Vegetarian Keto Diet Plan

How to Lose Weight Eating Healthy and Tasty Food

Maya Bryce

Disclaimer Notice:

Please note the information contained within this document is for educational and entertainment purposes only. All effort has been executed to present accurate, up to date, reliable, complete information. No warranties of any kind are declared or implied. Readers acknowledge that the author is not engaged in the rendering of legal, financial, medical or professional advice. The content within this book has been derived from various sources. Please consult a licensed professional before attempting any techniques outlined in this book.

By reading this document, the reader agrees that under no circumstances is the author responsible for any losses, direct or indirect, that are incurred as a result of the use of the information contained within this document, including, but not limited to, errors, omissions, or inaccuracies.

Table of Contents

Introduction

The vegetarian ketogenic diet changed my life.

This is a statement you might have heard before, but honestly, the introduction of both of these eating styles turned my eating habits around for the better, and better yet, they have aided me in losing the unwanted weight, which had been with me since childhood.

As someone who has struggled with weight loss most of my life, the constantly inflating belly, jiggling arms, and jean-ruining rubbing thighs are hauntingly familiar to me. Another familiar struggle is accepting that second offer of cake, consuming the extra slice of pizza because no one else will, and standing in the candy aisle at grocery stores deciding between a chocolate bar or leaving the aisle to buy some household goods that are actually needed at home.

The above-mentioned struggles and many others were part of my life for a long time until shrugging and laughing about my weight could no longer hide the fact that there was seriously something wrong with my eating habits.

Two of the first things that needed to change though were my thoughts and beliefs around weight loss and healthy eating. There were some fallacious ideas about myself that were constantly swimming around my head, which were often the cause of me not being able to fully commit to or complete a diet. My biggest misconception was believing there was a quick and easy way to lose weight. Although, it did finally dawn on me that there was no quick and easy fix to shedding those extra pounds.

Another one of my deterring thoughts was believing there was nothing wrong with my weight or eating habits. However, my constant discomfort with my body and the fact that my after three months new clothes got too tight clearly showed me that was not the truth. There was also the most backward and humiliating thought of all: physical exercise was merely a suggestion. Nonetheless, it soon became clear to me that physical exercise was one of the best ways to burn more calories than you consumed.

The vegetarian lifestyle had been part of my life for years before my weight became an issue and the ketogenic diet came onto the scene. Becoming a vegetarian was an eating style that came with new friends in my life who were either vegetarians or vegans. They did not force their lifestyle on me or trash-talk meat, but it was one of those 'show me your friends and I will show you your future' sort of scenarios. Although, I did not commit to the diet until some research and some eye-opening documentaries were undertaken, which taught me that meat wasn't the 'big cheese' everyone made it out to be. After that, it was easy to commit to the diet and meat was not a food that I missed in my life. However, there was more weight gain than loss because to substitute for the lack of meat and filling meals, my intake of vegetarian/vegan-friendly carbs and sugars increased.

Eventually though, the effect these carbs and sugars had become evident and cutting down my intake and going for 45-minute walks seemed like the solution; however, it wasn't until the ketogenic diet that everything really began to change.

As a vegetarian, you already practice watching what you eat but that is only with meat or some dairy products; the ketogenic diet is on another level, and the combination of both of these diets results in you eating healthier and less.

Nevertheless, once my combination of both of these eating styles began, there was no turning back. Another great thing was that working out became a regular routine in my life; the 45 minutes walks turned to intense cardio workouts that my body truly enjoyed. Eventually, as the weeks and months went by, my clothes became loose and baggy, the flat stomach I woke up to in the mornings remained intact even after breakfast, lunch, and dinner, and everything stayed where it is supposed to and these are the results that have kept me eating healthy and maintaining my new figure.

The Vegetarian Keto Diet Plan

Every person is different and one way does not always suit everyone, which is why the *Vegetarian Keto Diet Plan: How to Lose Weight Eating Healthy and Tasty Food* was written as a guide for all vegetarians seeking to implement the effects of the ketogenic diet into their lives.

If you've been looking for information about how to incorporate keto into you vegetarian lifestyle (or perhaps you want to make a complete switch to both keto and vegetarianism), then look no further as you will learn all about:

- What are the vegetarian and keto diets with the pros and cons to following this lifestyle

- Myths related to keto so you know what you are in for and what to expect

- Steps to follow to get you started on this new journey

- How to lose weight on the vegetarian keto diet

- Vegetarian keto-friendly foods you may eat (as well as the foods to avoid)

Tasty recipes you and your family can enjoy!

We want you to have a clear understanding about the vegetarian keto diet, attain progressive beliefs and thoughts that will only launch you upward and forward in your weight loss journey, and the ability to confidently state you know exactly what to do to lose weight, eating healthy vegetarian food the keto way.

Chapter 1: The Keto Diet & the Vegetarian Diet

The vegetarian keto diet is a combination of the ketogenic diet and the vegetarian diet. There is still some debate around the effects of the ketogenic diet but the same debate usually takes place around the vegetarian diet, and many of you reading this guide will be very aware there will always be someone saying something discouraging about eating styles that require you to cut out what the rest of the population considers to be 'essential' foods.

At the end of the day, if a life with a minuscule amount of carbs is something you can commit to, then you can make the ketogenic diet a permanent diet in your life. However, if you cannot bear to be without carbs, then we recommend you only use the ketogenic diet for three to maybe six months before returning to an everyday vegetarian diet. We will now be discussing the vegetarian and ketogenic diet at their core so we can better understand how these two diets can work together.

The Ketogenic Diet

The everyday diet consists of macronutrients.

And macronutrients or macros are our sources of nutrients; they are what we count when calculating calories and these macros are carbohydrates, fat, and protein. The recommended diet the majority of us grew up on consists of a high carb intake, a moderate intake of protein, and very low fat intake, and this is the diet that best meets our nutritional needs. However, most people's diets consist of a high fat, high carb, and even high protein intake, which is due to the fact that a lot of people can't afford to eat healthier, don't have the time to eat healthier, or they eat whatever because at least they ate something.

The ketogenic diet is good at halting this kind of unhealthy eating because on keto you are encouraged to consume more fats, moderate protein, and much fewer carbs. However, the suggested fats you should consume on the ketogenic diet are the good kinds of fat, good kinds of (low) carbs, and the good kinds of protein.

No sugary or starchy fats and carbs are to be found here.

What the ketogenic diet triggers is ketosis, which is a metabolic state that occurs in the body when the body is forced to burn fat for energy instead of carbohydrates. Carbohydrates are the regular fuel source for the body and glucose, which is produced by carbohydrates, is the default fuel for the brain. During ketosis, though, both the brain and body burn fat for energy, which is how you can burn fat (both the excess your body has stored and from dietary sources) and lose weight while you follow the keto diet.

When you are on the ketogenic diet, you are encouraged to consume foods, and you earn your calories through a diet that is high in fat, moderate in protein, and low in carbohydrates. Essentially, you must completely cut out all foods high in carbohydrates (grains, sugar, starch, etc.) from your diet, and invite good fats (avocados, olive oil, non-starchy vegetables, etc.) into your diet.

There are eight kinds of ketogenic diets. The standard ketogenic diet is the most common and is the basis for most, if not all, the other kinds of keto diets people follow.

#1. Standard Ketogenic Diet (SKD)

As the most common type of ketogenic diet, you can consume up to 20 to 50 grams of carbohydrates, 40 to 60 grams of protein, and 165 grams of fat. However, there is no set limit for fat because most of our calories should come from our fat intake so take the fat intake here as a suggestion.

#2. Very-Low-Carb Ketogenic Diet (VLCKD)

The very-low-carb ketogenic refers to a standard ketogenic diet but the diet consists of lower carb intake. On this diet, many people restrict their daily intake of carbs to between 20 and 30 grams.

#3. Well-Formulated Ketogenic Diet (WFKD)

The diet is similar to the *standard ketogenic diet* but in this instance, the macronutrients of fat, protein, and carbohydrates are identical to the ratios of the standard ketogenic diet. With this form of keto, there is a higher chance of ketosis taking place in the body. With

WFKD you have to stick to the set and recommended amounts of fat (165 grams), protein (40 grams), and carbs (20 grams). There is a set limit to fat.

#4. MCT Ketogenic Diet

The MCT ketogenic diet is based on the SKD, but the diet uses MCT oils to create 60% of the fats that will be burnt by the body. MCTs create more ketones per ounce of fat than the long-chain triglycerides, which are found in the standard everyday diet. Using MCT oils in your ketogenic diet ensures you will maintain ketosis and, at the same time, be able to eat more carbohydrates and protein. Consuming too much MCTs, especially on an inconsistent and unbalanced diet, can result in an upset stomach.

#5. Calorie-Restricted Ketogenic Diet

The calorie-restricted ketogenic diet restricts calories to a set amount. For women, 2,000 calories are the recommended maximum number of calories, and the recommended maximum calorie intake for men is 2,500. However, this keto diet could restrict your calorie intake to the minimum amount which is 1,200 calories.

#6. Cyclical Ketogenic Diet (CKD)

Another name for the cyclical ketogenic diet is the carb back-loading diet.

This is the keto diet that is recommended for athletes. Naturally, the diet allows athletes to enjoy a higher concentration of carbohydrates two days out of the week, which allows them to regain the glycogen in their muscles that was lost because of their intense training and working out schedules.

#7. Targeted Ketogenic Diet (TKD)

A combination of the standard ketogenic diet and the cyclical ketogenic diet is what the targeted ketogenic diet consists of. Basically, the diet allows you to consume more carbohydrates, but only on the days you exercise.

#8. High-Protein Ketogenic Diet

The high-protein ketogenic diet was created to assist individuals who need to lose weight for health reasons. The diet is based on the standard ketogenic diet and the diet consists of 35% protein, 60% fat, and 5% carbs.

The History of the Ketogenic Diet

Back in the 1920s and 1930s, the ketogenic diet was created and used to treat adults and children with epilepsy. Although, it is said the diet was temporarily abandoned when anticonvulsant therapies were introduced. On the other hand, the new medications failed to achieve the same astounding results as the ketogenic diet —especially in children, and so the ketogenic diet was reintroduced shortly after this assessment was made.

It seems that three individuals partook in the discovery of the keto diet.

Rollin Woodyatt was the endocrinologist who discovered that three kinds of ketone bodies—acetone, beta-hydroxybutyrate, and acetoacetate—were generated in the liver as a result of starvation or a high in fat and low in carb diet.

However, it was Russel Wilder of the Mayo Clinic who named the above-mentioned reaction in the body, discovered by Woodyatt, the ketogenic diet. And it was Peter Huttenlocher who first altered the keto diet so patients on the treatment could consume more protein and carbohydrates. Huttenlocher was able to make this alternation by suggesting that 60% of his patients' fat intake be gained mostly from MCT oils.

The Advantages of the Ketogenic Diet

#1. Weight Loss

With the ketogenic diet, the body enters a state of ketosis, and as a result, more ketones are created in the body. The ketones become the main source of energy for both the body and the brain. Usually, the brain burns the glucose from carbohydrates for energy and the body burns carbohydrates for energy. However, on the keto diet, the body and the brain burn fat for energy, so no excess fat is stored, and that results in weight loss.

#2. Epilepsy

As we have mentioned, the ketogenic was created as a therapeutic treatment for children and adults with epilepsy. The treatment was shortly abandoned but reintroduced to treat children who experienced epileptic seizures.

#3. Type 2 Diabetes

The low carb requirement of the ketogenic diet strongly impacts glucose concentrations, and it tends to lower glucose over time. Although, if you are a type 2 diabetic, we suggest that you consult with your doctor first before using the ketogenic diet as a solution.

#4. Cancer

There are not a lot of studies in regard to the advantages keto has on cancer, but according to Satterthwaite (2018, p. 134):

> The Warburg effect has established that tumour cells can break down glucose much faster (specifically 200x faster) compared to typical cells. The theory is that by 'starving' tumour cells of glucose, you can inhibit their growth and help prevent cancer.

The Disadvantages of the Ketogenic

Diet

#1. Keto Flu

The symptoms of the keto flu are constipation, fatigue, 'foggy brain', headaches, hunger, and irritability. The keto flu usually occurs at the start of the ketogenic diet (during the first week or two), and is due to the change in your diet; that is, cutting carbohydrates from your diet. Our suggestion is you remain well-rested and hydrated during the course of the diet to avoid and minimize your symptoms. Although, it is possible to avoid the keto flu by taking things slowly, as in changing your diet little by little instead of all at once.

#2. Nutrient Deficiencies

Nutrients are essential in any diet and for the body to function the way it should. We suggest that you follow the directions in this guide and only make alterations when you are certain you will not be cutting any needed nutrients out of your diet.

#3. Gut Health

Due to the lack of fiber and certain fruits in the keto diet, you might have issues in terms of being regular. There are other keto-friendly foods that offer you the needed amount of fiber, but we suggest you also remember to drink water along with following a balanced diet.

#4. Obedience

Maintaining any diet takes commitment, and dieting is occasionally easier said than done. With this diet, you will need to remain focused as not to self-sabotage by consuming the incorrect foods or giving up. We suggest you commit what is required of you to heart, remember the reason why you are doing this, and adhere to the guidelines written in this guide to assist you.

The Vegetarian Diet

The vegetarian diet—vegetarianism—is a diet that is meat, fish, and fowl flesh free. Mostly, we know vegetarians as environmentalists and individuals who are active in the fight regarding animal cruelty. There are only a few vegetarians —when asked— who are vegetarians purely for the health benefits.

Vegetarianism consists of about seven categories, but there are three kinds of vegetarian diets that are not considered to be "true" vegetarian.

Not True Vegetarian Diets

#1. Pescatarian

Pescatarians are individuals who occasionally consume fish and other seafoods but they do not consume any other animal flesh and some do not even consume animal by-products.

#2. Pollotarian

Pollotarians are people committed to the vegetarian diet but they often consume chicken and other poultry products, but they do not eat red or white meat.

#3. Flexitarian

Flexitarians live on a mostly plant-based diet but they occasionally consume meat, although they try to limit their meat intake when they can.

True Vegetarian Diets

On the other hand, the kinds of vegetarian diets that are considered to be the "proper" are:

#1. Veganism

Yes, veganism is a branch on the vegetarian tree.

The Vegetarian Society was first formed in England in the year 1847. However, it was only in 1944 that a man named Donald Watson coined the term vegan. He concluded that vegan would be used for vegetarians who did not consume eggs, meat, or animal by-products.

#2. Lacto Vegetarianism

Lacto vegetarians are vegetarians who do not consume any sort of animal flesh or eggs, but they use animal by-products like milk, cheese, and yogurt.

#3. Ovo Vegetarianism

The only animal by-product that ovo vegetarians consume are eggs. Ovo vegetarians do not consume red meat, white meat, fish, fowl, or any dairy products.

#4. Lacto-Ovo Vegetarianism

The most common vegetarian is a lacto-ovo vegetarian. These individuals do not consume red meat, white meat, fish, and fowl, but their veggie diet does include dairy products and eggs.

The History of the Vegetarian Diet

Historically, the vegetarian diet used to be known as the Pythagorean Diet. Yes, we are talking about the same Ancient Geek philosopher we learned about in geometry. Pythagoras was known as the father of vegetarianism for centuries, encouraging other like-minded individuals to partake in the same diet. However, in the mid-1800s, with the introduction of the Vegetarian Society in England, the Pythagorean Diet became known as the Vegetarian Diet.

Anthropologists state the vegetarian diet was popular long before Pythagoras, and they agree that the prehistoric humans' diet largely consisted of plants because plants cannot run away. Originally, the vegetarian diet was practiced for religious or ethical reasons (animal rights, etc.) However, today it is also practiced for health reasons.

The Advantages of the Vegetarian Diet

#1. Reduced Risk to Diseases

On a proper vegetarian diet, you are advised to consume whole grains, legumes, fruits, vegetables, nuts, and seeds, because these are the kinds of food packed with vitamins and minerals. The vitamins and minerals in these foods boost your health and reduce the risk of cardiovascular and gallstone disease.

#2. Prolonged Life

Certified medical practitioners have studied the link between plant-based diets and living longer, and the findings are fairly positive. Although, mindful eating, meditation and yoga, and regular exercise may play a major role in this advantage.

#3. Weight Control

It is said that plant-based diets are linked to weight loss, and that could be because we may consume less calories on a plant-based diet.

#4. Complete Nutrition

Studies have shown that it is easier to receive most of your macro and micronutrients on the vegetarian diet than on the vegan diet. Although there are some concerns regarding nutritional deficiencies on a vegetarian diet, there are more foods in the vegetarian diet that can supply you with those much-needed nutrients.

The Disadvantages of the Vegetarian Diet

#1. Nutrient Deficiencies

Vitamin B12, vitamin D, omega-3 fatty acids, calcium, and zinc are known as the vitamins that are lacking in a vegetarian diet, but sufficient nutrition can still be received through a proper and balanced vegetarian diet.

#2. Fewer Options

The vegetarian diet can be limiting at first because individuals cut out meat, seafood, and some other animal products. New vegetarians eventually learn the ropes to the vegetarian diet and their minds are opened to the healthy and tasty options and possibilities available to them.

#4. Inconvenient

The vegetarian diet can be inconvenient and time consuming with all the standing in grocery store isles reading the ingredients and checking the nutrition, minerals, and vitamins before throwing the food in your shopping cart. The same time-consuming processes can occur at restaurants and social gatherings. However, when you learn the ropes, you will become familiar with the restaurants that cater to your needs and you will be confident enough to bring your own vegetarian-friendly foods to social gatherings.

#4. Chemicals

Fruits, vegetables, and grains are often farmed using pesticides and herbicides, and the concern in the health community is that vegetarians may be more exposed to these chemicals because of their diet. The solution to this concern is to buy organic foods while the cheaper solution consists of carefully washing all the fruits and vegetables you buy and consume.

The Bottom Line

The ketogenic diet and the vegetarian diet have their differences.

Firstly, the ketogenic diet was basically created to work as a therapeutic treatment while the vegetarian diet was adopted for either religious or ethical reasons, and today the vegetarian diet seems to be more popular because of the diet's ethical background.

Secondly, the ketogenic diet focuses on limiting your intake of carbohydrates and increasing your intake of keto-friendly fats. The vegetarian diet, on the other hand, focuses on cutting or, for some vegetarians, limiting your intake of animal flesh and animal by-products.

Lastly, we can say the keto diet promotes ketosis, which is a metabolic state in the body that promotes ketones that assist you in burning fat and, thus, losing weight, while the vegetarian diet may consist of fewer calories than the regular everyday diet, which is how the vegetarian diet promotes weight loss.

There are three things these diets have in common, which is:

Firstly, the ketogenic diet and the vegetarian diet are considered to be healthy diets, and some even consider vegetarianism to be one of the healthiest diets in the world today.

Secondly, the keto diet and the vegetarian diet assist individuals in losing weight.

Lastly, the ketogenic diet and the vegetarian diet are helpful in fighting against long-term ailments such as cancer, diabetes, and cardiovascular issues.

The effects of the ketogenic and the vegetarian diets are pretty impressive. Both diets require practice and commitment, and you can really learn to be conscious about what foods you are putting in your body. Through the information in this chapter we trust you fully now understand exactly how you can learn to eat healthier and effectively lose weight on the vegetarian keto diet.

Our next chapter is packed with information about the steps you will need to take to implement the combination of these diets into your life, so we encourage you to read on, and we trust you will truly be encouraged with the next chapter.

Chapter 2: How to Get Started on the Vegetarian Keto Diet

You learned all about what the keto and vegetarian diets are in the previous chapter and may now wonder how you can combine these two. Clark (2020, p. 133) defines the vegetarian keto diet well:

> The simplest definition of the vegetarian ketogenic diet is a diet free of meat, fish, and fowl flesh that restricts carbohydrates. By eating in this way, we can reap all the benefits of the ketogenic diet while reducing our carbon footprint, decreasing animal abuse, and improving health.

Usually the biggest issues with starting a diet is the uncertainty, which could then lead you to make up excuses as to why you cannot commit fully to this diet change. When the rules are not entirely clear, we struggle to remain focused or enthusiastic about our new diet. We second-guess what we can eat, what we cannot eat, and how much we are allowed to consume during the diet all together, not to mention when something unexpected arises—how then to best deal with that and stay on your diet? And when we start to feel faint, we ask if certain activities—usually exercise —are allowed on the diet or if we are doing something wrong. Although, if you are feeling faint you might be doing something wrong or pushing too hard. Nonetheless, all the uncertainty and incorrect information leads to things like yo-yo dieting and, soon enough, we return to the 'comfortable' arms of our bad habits.

And worst of all, you gain all the weight back plus extra!

So, we recommend that you think about and even write out your intentions with this diet, and think about why you want to lose weight or eat healthier; it may sound silly, but writing things down is like talking out loud to yourself. Also write down the other diets you may have tried and why they didn't work out— more often than not the problem is in the mind. Once you write down the reason why you gave up, you can determine a path that would be solid for you. Maybe you gave up because you weren't seeing results, but everything takes time and every change consists of some struggles at the start.

Be kind and patient with yourself because you are trying something you have never tried before. We did not come walking straight out of our mother's womb, so why do we believe we can learn or develop a new habit on our first day? The first day is usually the toughest and every day after that is not always any better but eventually you will get the hang of things.

Write down your concerns, intentions, and any questions you may have, and hopefully we will answer most if not every one of your questions in this chapter.

In this chapter we look at the myths you might have heard about the ketogenic diet, tell you exactly what else you could do to lose weight on the vegetarian keto diet, and everything you need to know and consider before getting started with this lifestyle change.

Myths of the Ketogenic Diet

There are misconceptions we may have about the ketogenic diet.

Some of you may believe this is the ultimate diet to lose weight loss; however, that is not true because the reality is that the keto diet is not for everyone. There may also be some who may believe this is an unhealthy and unsafe diet—but again then people said (and still say!) the same thing about vegetarianism. If you already follow a vegetarian diet, you know it is healthy and you get all the nutrients you need The same way that there are incorrect ideas about the vegetarian diet, there is also incorrect information about the ketogenic diet. We'll look at these below so you will have the facts at hand.

#1. The Official Weight Loss Diet

Weight loss on the keto diet is possible most of all because of the person and not entirely because of the diet itself. The myth is that the ketogenic diet is the end-all-and-be-all diet, but this diet does not work for everyone because every individual does have different dietary needs.

Although, there are alterations that can be made or different variations of the diet can be tried like the different types of keto diets you learned about in our first chapter, but this diet does not always work in the same way for everyone.

The thing to do is experiment with the ketogenic diet and see what works best for you, but again, we lose weight when we are able to burn more calories than we are able to consume.

#2. Keto-Friendly Food & Sweeteners

When it comes to what you can and cannot eat on the ketogenic diet, people are still confused. There are either too few options or too many expensive alternatives, and then because fruits have too much sugar and vegetables have too many carbs some tend to believe these are the foods they should cut out during the ketogenic diet journey.

You should not cut out fruits and vegetables, especially the ones that are low in carbs and high in fiber—the latter especially is beneficial if you suffer from constipation.

Our other recommendation is that you remain focused on real food—so unprocessed as these usually contain all the extra and hidden carbs you want to avoid. Where possible, read the nutritional labels of the foods you buy and/or measure and calculate how much you can consume while still staying within the keto recommendations for carbs, protein, and fat.

Then there is the confusion and the debate about sweeteners.

One half says that sweeteners are the 'gateway' sticky sweet substance that could lead you back to carbs and unhealthy fats, thus throwing you off your keto lifestyle. The other half argues that they are more controlled than that, and if it weren't for the sweeteners, those keto-followers would not be able to comfortably commit to the diet.

Both are right because sweeteners can lead your body to have sugar cravings, but at the same time, sweeteners offer those on the diet the option of sweet, healthy treats to curb their cravings for non-keto-friendly food.

#3. Fat & Ketosis

Ketosis occurs in the body when the body has to burn fat instead of carbs for fuel, and this is a statement that leads some to believe that if they are not losing weight, it is because they are not consuming enough fats.

> One of the reasons keto diets work so well for weight loss is that they lower insulin levels and allow you to easily access your own fat stores for energy. This way of eating also helps you take in fewer calories by providing natural appetite suppression. (Spritzler, 2019, p. 136)

The solution here is to eat a little more protein, especially if you are consuming a less than moderate amount of this macro. The ketogenic diet does not consist of all the fats that we know and usually love but rather the healthy fats like olive oil, avocados, etc.

Do not make the mistake of consuming excessive amounts of fat without checking if they are heart-healthy and keto-friendly fats. Although, if you are still not losing weight after making these alterations, then try changing up your intake, the times that you eat, or try increasing your workout time or level of intensity.

#4. Yo-Yo Ketosis

Another misconception is that you can go back and forth on the ketogenic diet and be alright, which is a myth that is probably part of every diet and is so untrue.

Given the starting side-effects (keto flu, constipation, etc.) of the ketogenic diet, why would you even want to go back and forth? Once you are on the diet, stick to it, and if you are only temporarily on the diet, then stick to the diet until it comes time to end the diet. Also, when transitioning back to carbs, do so wisely and little-by-little to keep from overindulging and gaining back the pounds.

During the diet, you should wonder about the sort of healthy eating habits you would want to adopt into your life. Are you going to eat three times a day or five times a day? Are you going to eat all the carbs you missed during the diet or are you cutting some carbs out of your life for good? Are you still going to be drinking the correct amount of water or are you going straight back for fruit juices and all the other beverages that you might have missed during the ketogenic diet?

The ketogenic diet is an ideal time to ponder on these sorts of changes, a great way to practice healthy eating, and your chance to learn about limiting your calorie intake.

#5. Regarding Proteins

There are two misconceptions here; the first being that the ketogenic diet is all about protein, which it is not. The ketogenic diet is a low-carb, high-fat, and moderate protein diet. The second misconception is that too much protein can deter weight loss, but again, this is not true.

You should eat a moderate and the recommended (because our bodies are different) amount of protein. Too much protein can be turned to glucose and lead you to fall out of ketosis, while too little protein can lead to a larger appetite, decreased metabolic rate, and cause you to lose muscle mass.

Steps to the Ketogenic Diet

#1. Understand the Ketogenic Diet

As you've learned (and we delve a little deeper into this here), the keto diet recommends a daily macro intake of high fats, low carbs, and moderate protein (instead of the usual high carb, low fat, and moderate protein diet most people follow). With the restricted intake of carbs, the body is forced to burn fat instead of carbohydrates and ketones are generated in the body—in your liver, to be exact—and your body and brain use the ketones as their new source of energy.

However, this does not mean you can eat all the healthy fats in the world and still be burning fat, because your calories intake still matters.

On keto, weight loss is initially achieved from the water weight you lose due to the depletion of glycogen. Beyond that, your body burns both dietary and body fat, meaning that your excess fat stores are used, and this helps aid in weight loss. Further, due to the kinds of keto-friendly meals you will prepare, you will feel more satiated, leading you to feel fuller for longer, and thus, eat less or consume fewer calories.

The ketogenic diet encourages you to consume healthy fats and no starchy carbohydrates. Essentially, the ketogenic diet encourages you to practice a strict and healthy diet, which is why it works so well for so many individuals.

#2. Keto-Friendly Food

The next thing to do after knowing what to focus on is to learn about keto foods, which ones you can consume, which ones to avoid entirely, and which ones you can have occasionally.

On the ketogenic diet, the consumption suggestion we are given is that 55% to 60% of your daily meals should be fats and 5% to 10% should be carbs, and the remainder goes to protein. Although, again, everyone is different and needs certain amounts of macros, which is why we suggest you talk to a medically licensed dietician if you are ever unsure about how this restrictive diet will work for you.

However, simply put, you should only consume keto-friendly foods. Our next chapter will tell you more about the foods you can eat, cannot eat, and what you should be shopping for.

#3. Fatty Relationship

One of the things to do before committing to this diet is to consider your relationship with fat. As keto is the opposite of what you may be used to (high carb, low fat), you must look at your relationship with fat as you will be consuming much more of this. We have all heard that fat is bad for us, that fat clogs up our arteries to kill us, and as a result, a number of people are afraid of fat.

However, that is untrue, especially if you stick to healthy fats, which include avocados, certain nuts, nut butters, and olive oil (and some other options). If you happen to be the sort of person who is afraid of donuts and fries, that is okay, because those are not recommended on this diet and you can continue to stay away from those unhealthy foods.

If you are afraid of consuming even healthy fats (and in larger quantities), we recommend that you and fat become introduced quickly or at a pace you are comfortable with. How about reading up on some studies that illustrate the health benefits healthy fats have in store for you to get you started?

#4. Calculator

The three macronutrients are carbs, fats, and protein. Neither one of these macros should ever be completely cut out of your diet because then you may experience a nutrient deficiency, and this may lead to other illnesses. The low carbs you consume on keto offer you much-needed fiber, protein repairs the body, and fats suppress your appetite, plus, it is your main source of energy on keto.

When you start out on keto, you may need to learn to start tracking the number of macros you consume, and you do this by knowing how many calories you need. There are apps (MyFitnessPal, Cronometer, MyMacros+) that you can download on

hone or other smart device to
your calorie intake and your
macros; however, you could also
calculate your macros manually:

As you might remember, on the
standard American diet, people
consume 45% to 60% of their calories
from carbohydrate sources, 20% to 35%
from fats, and the remainder from
protein. On the ketogenic diet though,
the ratios are as follows

- 5% to 10% from carbs
- 60% to 75% from fat
- 15% to 30% from protein

On a standard 2,000-calorie keto diet,
here is how you can calculate how many
grams of each macro you can consume
per day. An important note: carbs and
protein have 4 calories per gram, while
fats have 9 calories per gram.

When we calculate the carbs: 2,000 x
0.05 = 100 carb calories. Divide this by
4 = 25 grams of carbs, which is your
carb intake for the day, every day.

When we calculate the fats: 2,000 x 0.65 = 1,300 fat calories, divided by 9 = 144.44 grams of fat, which is your fat intake for the day, every day.

Lastly, we calculate the protein: 2,000 x 0.20 = 400 protein calories, divided by 4 = 100 grams of protein, which is your fat intake for the day, every day.

Until the diet becomes second nature, we recommend you only eat what you calculate and measure. Although this may seem like an inconvenience, it will certainly assist you in watching what you eat and will be better for you in general in the long run. This way, you can then also more easily make adjustments if you aren't losing weight or experience side effects.

#5. Clean House

Okay, so having only keto-friendly foods in your house is easier said than done.

You might be unsure which foods are keto-friendly and you may assume that all fruits and vegetables are the correct foods to be eating on a vegetarian keto diet but that is simply not true (more info on this coming soon so you know exactly what foods to keep, what to throw out, and what to add to your shopping list).

We suggest getting rid of any foods that may lead you astray, especially before you start the diet to help you exert control and stay on track. This is also helpful until you learn what to do when you have cravings or they disappear. Remember that we only experience cravings when our body wants a certain nutrient or mineral. Whatever your craving may be, there is a keto-friendly substitute that exists.

#6. Goals, Family, & Spotters

Another step to take towards the keto diet is considering your goals, sharing your plans with your family or friends, and getting someone to tag along or, at the very least, to 'spot' you.

Ask yourself now what do you want to accomplish with this diet and what do you see as the end result of your hard work, time, and sacrifices. You have to be realistic with your goals. Write down what you want to see, what habits you may want to implement in your life, and imagine the way you see yourself achieving your set goals. When we say things out loud, we often find the plot holes in our ideas and then we can make alterations where needed.

The reasons you chose to embark on this vegetarian keto journey are only known to you, but teamwork makes the dream work, so we suggest you talk to a family member or friends about your reasons. You could even ask a friend or a relative —one practiced in being committed and who would only motivate you to keep going—to tag along with you on the diet. Seriously, though, be wise and honest with yourself because you don't want to pick the friend who would sit with you on the couch and eat ice-cream with you on the days you feel like giving up; rather ask the friend who would remind you of your goals and the reasons giving up is not the answer.

If no one is willing to join you, you could ask them to be spotters, check on you every now and then, and you can go to them when you are having a hard time. Although, the best person to push you forward is you, so do the basic thing and get yourself a mantra and stick it above your mirror.

#7. Determination

Do not use your heart for this instead use your head.

Going into something just because it feels like the good thing or the right thing hardly guarantees results. You need to change your thinking and make the decision every day to persevere and remain determined, which is the right attitude to have.

Entering the diet with a goal in mind can only take you so far if you have the wrong attitude. You will need to adopt a 'will-do' attitude and remain committed and focused, even on the difficult days. You made an agreement with yourself to commit for a certain number of weeks or months and you cannot give up.

Are you ready to be totally and fully committed?

Okay, maybe committed is a big word because everything takes practice. There will be mistakes along the way, mistakes are excellent learning opportunities, and remembering everything you can and cannot do can be rather daunting at first. Although, with keto flu, we suggest you start this diet during a slow—not much going on—sort of week or over a long and chilled weekend.

During the first week, try to store only keto-friendly foods in the house, avoid that social gathering if you know you will be stuffing your face with processed foods by the end of the night, plan and calculate all your meals, and hydrate.

You could seriously use this diet as a chance to make some changes in your life. Note the bad habits that could be draining you or causing you to be unfocused about the other goals you want in your life. During this diet, you need to be tough on yourself and practice discipline.

We understand that some days are harder than others, and on those days, we recommend that you be honest with your spotter or someone who will understand. Talking things out can help you remember why keto-unfriendly food is a bad idea, it can also remind you of your goals, and talking out loud means you are louder than the voice in your head telling you to throw in the towel.

#8. Consider the Future

There are still some debates about the effects that the ketogenic diet can have as a long-term diet, but as we mentioned in our firsts chapters the same debate is still going on regarding the various vegetarian diets. The diet can be long-term or short-term depending on the person, but if you cannot live comfortably with a low amount of carbs, then make this a short-term keto diet.

Either way, you should still consider life after the diet or once you've settled into things. What sort of eating habits do you want to have once the diet is over? How often do you want to be eating on a daily basis?? What foods are you never going back to again? What foods are you excited to invite back into your life?

During the diet, note what is working for you and what is not working for you. Avoid going right back to a typical American diet and gaining back all the weight you lost. Truly consider what changes you would want to see in your life after the completion of this diet.

Burning Unwanted Fat

Sometimes, losing weight on the keto diet does not happen for some people, and we will now discuss if that could be because the diet isn't for them or if it is because they are doing something wrong. We are going to focus more on the things you could be doing wrong though if you aren't burning fat on the ketogenic diet and entering into a state of ketosis.

We will discuss the symptoms of the ketosis first.

There are the obvious symptoms, and the most obvious would be the *keto flu*, which we discussed in the previous chapter. The keto flu is a symptom of a changing diet but that is not the only symptom of ketosis.

Bad breath would be the first symptom, which is caused by a ketone—acetone—that exits in the body through the urine and the breath. The release of this ketone causes your breath to take on a more fruity smell.

Weight loss would be a clear and obvious sign that you are in ketosis, although during the first week, the weight you lose is considered to be stored carbs and water. However, seeing weight loss in the first week is a regular occurrence, and seeing yourself losing one to two pounds a week is another regular occurrence of the diet.

Decreased appetite is another symptom, which means you won't get as hungry as you used to or as often. Researchers say that this loss of appetite could be ketones 'telling' your brain to reduce your appetite.

Restlessness is the last symptom we are going to mention that has to do with ketosis; you may experience sleepless nights during the early stages of ketosis, but once your body gets used to things, you could even sleep better than before.

There are other symptoms like increased ketones in the blood and breath, increased focus and energy, fatigue and lowered performance, and digestive issues. Remember that if you are not seeing changes in your weight, these could be reasons:

#1. You could be eating too many carbs. You are supposed to limit your carbs to 5% to 10%. If you started the diet at 10%

and you are not losing weight, then decrease your carb intake accordingly.

#2. You may not be eating foods that are not filled with enough nutrients or you may be snacking on high-calorie foods. We suggest that you stick to whole foods and stay away from processed and fast food because they do not have the nutrients that you need, plus they may contain too many carbs. Also, in regard to snacks, although they may help with hunger between meals, try to limit the amount of snacks you consume in a week. Snacks and desserts are extra calories you do not need.

#3. You have not created a calorie deficit and that is one big way to lose weight on the ketogenic diet. Tracking, calculating, and measuring your calories help you create a deficit and so does working out. You cannot expect to lose weight if you are not watching what you eat and working out. Being physically active is important in any sort of diet. You can't expect to lose weight from just the way you eat; remember, you need to be burning more calories than the number of calories you consume.

#4. Another reason for not losing weight could be undiagnosed medical issues (depression, hypothyroidism, and high insulin levels). You could have a doctor check you out for any of these and you can move on with the diet from there. Another issue that could cause you to remain at the same weight is your stress levels and lack of sleep. Chronic stress causes the body to store up fat, which is the cause of that bulging belly.

#5. There is a quote on Pinterest (n.d.) about weight lost:

> It takes 4 weeks for you to notice a change. It takes 8 weeks for your friends to notice. It takes 12 weeks for the rest of the world to notice a change. It takes one day to decide that you are enough.

This was true for me; it may, however, not be true for you but this sure helped me to remain focused, and it reminded me that everything—no matter how much you want it or push at it—takes time. You may not have realistic weight loss goals, which could cause you to believe that nothing is happening; losing one to two pounds a week is healthy and within the range of what most people lose in that time frame.

The Bottom Line

After putting together the lists of myths surrounding the ketogenic diet, the things to consider before getting started on your vegetarian ketogenic diet, and what else to consider if you are not burning fat, we felt that journaling your progress would be of great assistance to you.

Journaling is one way to organize your thoughts—we are well aware that our thoughts can make or break us during our journey to healthy eating and weight loss. Our cravings begin as a thought that runs through our mind on a loop until we lose all reason why stuffing our faces with freshly made bread or warm chocolate chip cookies is a bad idea.

At the start of your journal, you could write down the reasons you are on the diet—seriously, it is hard to remember the reasons you need to stay on track on those really difficult days. Write what you expect from the diet and then rewrite your expectations if they are not realistic. During those difficult days, try journaling your thoughts and feelings over melting into the couch and stuffing your face with all the carbs you can find around the house.

And one of the beneficial things about journaling is being able to look back on the pages of your journal on other hard days and you will be reminded of why you are on this diet and remember all the days where you overcame and see how exactly you were able to subdue your cravings with keto-friendly foods.

We understand that journaling is not always for every person and, if that is the case, then you could try doodling, recording voice notes, video journaling, or simply listing your thoughts and feelings without providing any context, as long as you are aware of where you are on your journey and where you want to be at the end.

Always be honest and patient with yourself.

We trust this guide is able to encourage, enlighten, and assist you in getting started on a vegetarian keto diet. Remember to always keep your head held high—no false confidence here—and remain focused on the goals you want to accomplish.

Lastly, we believe your steps will be sure and your food will be measured!

Chapter 3: Vegetarian Keto Foods

This guide is specifically designed for lacto-ovo vegetarians on the *standard ketogenic diet*, and so we will follow the keto daily recommendations of 165 grams of fat, 40 grams of carbohydrates, and 75 grams of protein. For non-vegetarians who may be interested in combining the ketogenic diet and the vegetarian diet to lose weight or any other reason, this vegetarian keto diet is a meat-free diet (no animal flesh) and meat is not included in the list of foods to be consumed while on this diet or in the recipes.

We advise that you be aware of hidden carbs and read the nutrition labels (especially on processed and pre-packaged foods), especially at the start of the diet until you can be sure that whatever you are eating is keto friendly.

Our suggestion is that you avoid sugar, grains, starch, trans fats and hydrogenated fats, certain fruits, low-fat foods, and certain vegetables at all costs. There is a list of prohibited food below; however, there are some that need their own mentions.

Alcohol should be avoided, and if you can't, then alcohol intake should be limited to only hard liquor (rum, vodka, gin, etc.), low carb beer, and wine. Another suggestion is to avoid snacking and desserts, because these meals could slow down your weight loss; therefore, snack and enjoy dessert at your own discretion. If you do intend to consume snacks (and it is always good to be prepared with snacks in case the hunger bug bites) and dessert, we have some recipes for you to try. In regard to condiments, we suggest making your own when possible because most condiments are not keto-friendly (due to the extra carbs). Permitted condiments include reduced sugar ketchup, yellow mustard, keto-friendly ranch dressing, low-carb mayonnaise, vinaigrette dressing, and soy sauce.

Sweeteners like honey are not allowed at all but there are sweeteners like Stevia, sucralose, erythritol, monk fruit, yacon syrup, and xylitol that are keto-friendly and are safe to use. Always remember to check those nutrition labels and avoid artificial sweeteners.

We have arranged our lists into two categories—*forbidden and allowed foods* — in a list from A to Z.

The Forbidden Foods for a Vegetarian Keto Diet

The following is a list of foods you should try to avoid at all times during the vegetarian ketogenic diet. These foods are on this list because they are too high in carbs, and this can easily kick you out of ketosis. However, some of the food on this to-be-avoided list can, at times, be consumed in moderate amounts.

- Agave. Apples. Apricots.
- Bananas. Barbecue Sauce. Beans. Beer. Beetroots. Black Beans. Bread. Brown Sugar. Buckwheat.
- Carrots. Cereal. Chickpeas. Cocktails. Cookies. Corn. Crackers.
- Energy Drinks.
- Granola. Grapefruit.
- Honey. Honey Mustard.
- Juice.
- Ketchup.
- Lentils.
- Maple Syrup. Margarine. Marinades. Melon.
- Oats. Oranges.
- Parsnips. Pasta. Peanuts. Peas. Plums. Potato Chips. Potatoes. Pretzels.
- Quinoa.
- Rice. Rye.

- Soda. Sports Drinks. Sweet Potatoes. Sweet Tea. Sweetened Salad Dressings.
- Wheat. White Sugar. Wine.
- Yams.

The Allowed Foods on the Vegetarian Keto Diet

Below is a list of foods you are allowed to consume on the ketogenic diet. Although, you should know that just because a food is permitted or has a low carb intake, does not mean you can eat as much of that food as you want.

- Aged Cheddar. Almond Butter. Almond Flour. Almonds.
- Baby Mushrooms. Blackberries. Blueberries. Brazil Nuts. Brie. Broccoli.

- Cabbage. Cauliflower. Chia Seed Meal. Coconut Flour. Cottage Cheese. Cream Cheese.
- Flaxseed Meal.
- Greek Yogurt. Green Beans. Green Bell Pepper.
- Half n' half. Hazelnuts. Heavy Cream.
- Macadamia Nuts. Mascarpone. Mayonnaise. Mozzarella.
- Parmesan. Pecans.
- Raspberries. Romaine Lettuce.
- Spinach.
- Tempeh. Tofu.
- Unsweetened Coconut.
- Yellow Onion.

The Weekly Grocery List

Listed below is everything you can purchase on the keto diet and these foods are vegetarian friendly. You can use this list as a basis of what to place in your shopping cart and what to leave behind. You can also determine your budget by going through this list to know what to buy. It would help if you planned your meals in advance to know what sort of food to always have in the house.

Beverages

- Almond milk
- Coconut milk
- Coffee
- Tea
- Water

Fruits

- Avocado
- Coconut
- Cranberries
- Lemon
- Lime
- Olives

- Raspberries
- Strawberries
- Tomatoes
- Watermelon

Vegetables

- Artichoke
- Arugula
- Asparagus
- Bell peppers
- Broccoli
- Cabbage
- Cauliflower
- Celery
- Collards
- Cucumbers
- Eggplant
- Garlic
- Lettuce
- Mushrooms
- Radishes
- Shallots
- Spinach
- Swiss chard

- Turnips
- Zucchini

The Fridge & Freezer Staples

- Apple cider vinegar
- Cauliflower rice
- Frozen berries
- Pickles
- Micro-greens
- Sauerkraut
- Sprouts
- Tempeh
- Tofu

Pantry Staples

- Almond flour
- Baking powder
- Baking soda
- Coconut flour
- Coconut milk (canned)
- Cocoa powder

- Dark chocolate (90%)
- Nutritional yeast
- Vanilla extract

Nuts & Seeds

- Almonds
- Brazil nuts
- Chia seeds
- Flax seeds
- Hazelnuts
- Hemp seeds
- Macadamia nuts
- Pecans
- Pumpkin seeds
- Sunflower seeds

Herbs & Spices

- Basil
- Cayenne Pepper
- Chili Powder
- Cilantro

- Cinnamon
- Cumin
- Oregano
- Parsley
- Rosemary
- Thyme

Nut & Seed Butters

- Almond butter
- Coconut butter
- Hazelnut butter
- Peanut butter
- Pecan butter
- Sunflower seed butter

Healthy Oils

- Almond oil
- Avocado oil
- Coconut oil
- Hazelnut oil
- Macadamia nut oil

- MCT oil
- Olive oil

Sauces & Condiments

- Horseradish
- Hot Sauce
- Ketchup (no sugar added)
- Mustard
- Relish (no sugar added)
- Salad Dressings (no sugar added)
- Sauerkraut (no sugar added)
- Worcestershire Sauce

Sweeteners

- Erythritol
- Monk fruit
- Stevia
- Sucralose
- Xylitol
- Yacon Syrup

The Bottom Line

We are well aware that too often the issue with dieting is the purchasing of the above-mentioned products, which can be an expensive endeavor, and this is why we suggest you budget or even save up before starting. However, there are ways to start keto on a tight budget.

We understand that even thinking about how to get started or where to get the best deals could discourage you from giving this diet a real go. Top tips to get started on keto even when you don't have a large budget includes:

- Buying the groceries that will last longer in bulk
- Always looking for sales and shopping online to get better deals
- Buying fruits and vegetables that are in season
- Choosing the frozen fruits and vegetables over the fresh ones

because they hold up better over long periods of time

- Planning your meals ahead of time so when you go to the store, you do not waste cash on food you think you need (and are not planned)
- Considering preparing your meals during the week in such a way that you will have leftovers that you can store for lunch the following day or dinner when you don't have time to cook.

Every person is different and, through the course of the diet, you will learn tips and tricks that work best for you. However, when it comes to cravings, we must think before we act; there are two things to consider:

Firstly, what is a keto-friendly substitute for what you are craving?

Secondly, is it the right time for you to be eating?

It sounds like a lot but take things at your own pace and try to learn one tip and trick at a time, as learning everything at once can be overwhelming. Through constant repetition and sticking to the vegetarian keto diet, you will learn to use these tips and tricks without even thinking about it.

Chapter 4: Keto-Friendly Fruits & Vegetables

Truthfully, for some of us—vegetarians—fruits and vegetables are our largest source of food, but because of the sugar in fruits and the carbs in vegetables, we are forced to remove some fruits and vegetables from our everyday diet if we want to follow keto.

Vegetables (especially those that grow underground) tend to have too much starch, fruits tend to have too much sugar, and together, they have too many calories that if consumed can cause you to fall out of ketosis. However, there are enough low-carb fruits and vegetables you can consume on the keto diet.

Keto-Friendly Fruits

Avocado

Nutrition Facts (100 grams)

Calories: 160

Fat: 15 grams

Carbohydrates: 9 grams

Protein: 2 grams

Originally, avocados come from south-central Mexico and are classified as a fruit even though the *botanically large berry* is used as a vegetable. The fruit is rich in vitamins, such as vitamin A, C, B-6, and magnesium.

Avocados are the most popular keto-friendly fruit out there, as they are included in so many of the recipes. They taste amazing, so it is totally understandable. Although, it is not only their taste that makes them so likable but also because they are rich in healthy fats.

Benefits of eating avocado include their ability to help combat heart disease and lower your cholesterol. Avos also improve insulin sensitivity, lower inflammation, and they contain more potassium than a banana (which is great, because you can't eat these yellow fruits while following keto).

At the end of the chapter, there is a wonderful *Keto Chocolate Ice Cream* recipe for you to try out, and the ice cream is made from avocados.

Blackberries

Nutrition Facts (100 grams)

Calories: 43

Fat: 0.5 grams

Carbohydrates: 10 grams

Protein: 1.4 grams

The blackberry comes from the Rosaceae family tree and is rich in vitamin A and C, calcium, iron, and magnesium. Blackberries are another keto-friendly fruit that you might not have thought about all that much, but you will be surprised to learn how much this little black fruit can do.

This fruit is rich in a number of vitamins that reduce inflammation, promote brain and motor function, healthy skin, and vitamins that slow the growth of cancer cells in the body.

Blackberries have also been used for years as a medicine, which is understandable given the fact that this fruit can do so much already on its own. Another amazing thing to note about blackberries is how rich they are in fiber, which means this fruit should be in great supply in your household at the start of your diet, because fiber can help with any gut issues you may have.

At the end of the chapter, there is a lovely blackberry inspired *Berry Pops* recipe that you can try out, which is another example of the tasty treats you can make with keto-friendly fruits.

Blueberries

Nutrition Facts (100 grams)

Calories: 57

Fat: 0.3 grams

Carbohydrates: 14 grams

Protein: 0.7 grams

Blueberries are native to North America, and are packed with vitamin C, vitamin A, iron, vitamin B-6, and magnesium. This is similar to the benefits of blackberries, which also promote healthy skin, brain and motor function, and your health in general.

Blueberries also assist in combating skin infections. However, blueberries contain the most carbs when compared to other keto-friendly berries, and so we suggest you limit your intake of this fruit.

Melons

Nutrition Facts (100 grams)

Calories: 30

Fat: 0,2 grams

Carbohydrates: 8 grams

Protein: 0,6 grams

Watermelons are farmed all over the world, but they originate from West Africa. The fruit contains vitamin A, vitamin C, and magnesium. The safest watermelons to have on the ketogenic diet is casaba melon, watermelon, cantaloupe, and honeydew melon, because they are low in carbs and have the least amount of sugar.

Honeydew melon fuels you throughout the day with its natural sugars, and it can boost your immune system, help keep your heart functioning the right way, and wash out toxins in the body that can cause illnesses.

Cantaloupe promotes healthy eye function, growth, and maintenance of cells in the body, as well as healthy teeth.

Watermelon, on the other hand, contains lycopene, which is an antioxidant that prevents cell damage and several types of cancer in the body. Other vitamins and minerals in the watermelon assist in boosting cardiovascular health.

Nevertheless, melon is another fruit you have to be careful with on the ketogenic diet; ensure you measure and calculate your intake of carbs.

Raspberries

Nutrition Facts (100 grams)

Calories: 53

Fat: 0,7 grams

Carbohydrates: 12 grams

Protein: 1,2 gram

Raspberries come from the Rubus plant, which is a plant of the rose family, and they are filled with vitamin C, calcium, iron, magnesium, and vitamin B-6. This tiny red fruit is also packed with antioxidants that fight against inflammation. Raspberries contain a high polyphenol content and this can help reduce blood pressure and prevent plaque building up in the arteries.

Starfruit

Nutrition Facts (100 grams)

Calories: 31

Fat: 0,3 grams

Carbohydrates: 7 grams

Protein: 1 gram

Averrhoa carambola is a tree that can be found in tropical sectors around the world and grows star fruit. Star fruit or carambola consists of vitamin C, magnesium, and vitamin A.

This fruit is keto-friendly. It looks like a lemon and bell pepper combo, and has a sweet and sour taste to it. The star fruit is anti-inflammatory and heart-friendly, regulates blood pressure, and promotes weight loss.

Strawberries

Nutrition Facts (100 grams)

Calories: 33

Fat: 0,3 grams

Carbohydrates: 8 grams

Protein: 0,7 grams

Strawberries is our second last fruit on this list. The fruit is grown and enjoyed on a world-wide scale, and it is classified as a hybrid species of the genus Fragaria. The strawberry is rich in vitamin C, iron, magnesium, and calcium.

Strawberries are beneficial when it comes to blood sugar levels, insulin levels, and in promoting insulin sensitivity. Although, be wise about how many strawberries you consume and how often you consume them because you don't want to risk falling out of ketosis.

Tomatoes

Nutrition Facts (100 grams)

Calories: 18

Fat: 0,2 grams

Carbohydrates: 3,9 grams

Protein: 0,9 grams

Originally, tomatoes came from western South America and Central America. Tomatoes are rich with vitamin C, potassium, folate, and vitamin K.

The tomato is a fruit used too often as a vegetable and not just in the ketogenic diet. There is also the antioxidant lycopene in tomatoes, the same antioxidant found in watermelons, and it promotes heart disease and cancer.

At the end of the chapter, there is a tasty *Tomato Soup* recipe you can try out and enjoy on those chilly winter nights.

Keto-Friendly Vegetables

When it comes to vegetables, the best and safest are the above ground vegetables. Underground vegetables generally contain too many carbs, especially potatoes and sweet potatoes, so say goodbye to those crispy fries and mashed potatoes.

Onions are another major no-no, but because we mainly stick to the spice (onion powder) and we do not generally consume all that many onions, they are permitted. However, it would be better to use scallions or green onions if you really need to use an onion in a recipe. Know and research your alternatives, especially if you are developing a non-ketogenic recipe into a vegetarian keto-friendly one.

Another recommendation is to stick to the red bell peppers as the green and yellow have a higher carb count. If you are ever unsure about which vegetables to pick, then always go for green and leafy ones.

We can summarize that above ground, green, and leafy vegetables are our safest bet. One exception is corn.

Asparagus

Nutrition Facts (100 grams)

Calories: 20

Fat: 0,1 grams

Carbohydrates: 3,9 grams

Protein: 2,2 grams

The young shoots of asparagus are used as spring vegetables. The vegetable contains vitamin A, vitamin C, iron, and vitamin B-6. Asparagus promotes blood clotting, bone health, cell growth, and DNA formation.

You can try baking and melting cheese over your asparagus, or you could roast or cook this vegetable and pair it with a keto-friendly sauce or other dinner meals.

Bell Pepper

Nutrition Facts (100 grams)

Calories: 31

Fat: 0.3 grams

Carbohydrates: 6 grams

Protein: 1 gram

Bell peppers come in a variety of colors, from green, orange, white, yellow, red, and purple. Bell peppers are packed with vitamin A, vitamin C, magnesium, and vitamin B-6, and the green bell peppers contain the lowest number of carbs.

You could stuff your peppers with a compatible ingredient of your choice or chop them up into your breakfast eggs or add color to your fried cauliflower rice recipe.

Broccoli

Nutrition Facts (100 grams)

Calories: 34

Fat: 0,4 grams

Carbohydrates: 7 grams

Protein: 2,8 grams

Broccoli is part of the cabbage family and filled with vitamin C, vitamin A, vitamin B-6, and magnesium. Broccoli is a fun green vegetable that can be steamed or roasted and/or covered in cheese. The vegetable is crunchy and filled with so much flavor.

There are several ways to enjoy broccoli but there is a *Roasted Broccoli* recipe for you to try out at the end of the chapter.

Cauliflower

Nutrition Facts (100 grams):

Calories: 25

Fat: 0,3 grams

Carbohydrates: 5 grams

Protein: 1,9 grams

Cauliflower is an annually grown plant, which is packed with vitamin C, vitamin B-6, and magnesium. The cauliflower is a vegetable you should always have in the house, because there are so many things you can make with cauliflower. You can use it as a rice and mash it or even chopped it into chicken-like bits. You can really play around with this vegetable.

There is a great *Hash Browns* recipe at the end of this chapter in which you can use your cauliflower.

Green Beans

Nutrition Facts (100 grams)

Calories: 31

Fat: 0,1 grams

Carbohydrates: 7 grams

Protein: 1,8 grams

Green beans are part of the bean family and are a source of vitamin C, vitamin B-6, magnesium, iron, and calcium. These veggies are good for your eyes, heart, and digestion.

Green beans are quite enjoyable and can be enjoyed as an excellent side-dish with any of your dinner meals; and they can be enjoyed steamed or roasted.

Lettuce

Nutrition Facts (100 grams)

Calories: 15

Fat: 0,2 grams

Carbohydrates: 2,9 grams

Protein: 1,4 grams

Lettuce is part of the daisy family and offers you vitamins like vitamin A, vitamin C, iron, calcium, vitamin B-6, and magnesium. This leafy hydrating vegetable is low in calories, promotes weight loss, and is packed with antioxidants.

There are different kinds of lettuce (iceberg, butter, radicchio, romaine, kale, and many others) you can use in your meals for crunch and for a heighted flavor, and yes, lettuces can be used for more than just salads.

Mushrooms

Nutrition Facts (100 grams)

Calories: 22

Fat: 0,3 grams

Carbohydrates: 3,3 grams

Protein: 3,1 grams

Mushrooms are classified as a fungus that is packed with vitamin C, iron, vitamin B-6, and magnesium. This veggie is an immune system booster and the antioxidants in the vegetable combat things like heart disease and cancer.

Mushrooms can be chopped and thrown in the frying pan, glazed with garlic sauce and paired with some bell peppers and eggs, or added to cauliflower rice for extra taste.

Spinach

Nutrition Facts (100 grams)

Calories: 23

Fat: 0,4 grams

Carbohydrates: 3,6 grams

Protein: 2,9 grams

Originally, this leafy green vegetable came from central and western Asia. Spinach is packed with calcium, magnesium, and vitamin A. This vegetable is low in carbs and high in nutrients, which makes it one of the best vegetables to always have around.

The best way to enjoy spinach is as a creamy side-dish, so check out the recipe at the end of this chapter, and add your own little twist to it if you want.

Zucchini

Nutrition Facts (100 grams)

Calories: 17

Fat: 0,3 grams

Carbohydrates: 3,1 grams

Protein: 1,2 grams

A zucchini is classified as a summertime squash. The cucumber-looking vegetable is filled with vitamin C, iron, vitamin B-6, and magnesium. Zucchini aid in weight loss and promote healthy digestion.

There are a number of recipes you can find that use zucchini on the vegetarian keto diet like fries and chips. You can grill, fry, and grate zucchini for use in your recipes.

Keto-Friendly Veggie & Fruit Recipes

Keto Chocolate Ice Cream

Keto Chocolate Ice Cream is the bittersweet ice cream that offers you the chance to indulge in a sweet but healthy treat.

Ensure that the ingredients you use are keto-friendly and that they are low in sugar.

The recipe below yields 6 servings. Although, you can alter it to one serving in case you are easily tempted to overindulge.

Note: if you do not have an ice cream maker, then no worries; our instructions below cover another way to still make this recipe.

Time: 12 hours

Serving Size: 1 bowl

Prep Time: 4 hours

Cook Time: 8 hours

Nutritional Facts/Info:

Calories: 216.17 grams

Carbs: 3.72 grams

Fat: 19.38 grams

Protein: 3.86 grams

Ingredients:

- 25 drops liquid Stevia
- 6 squares unsweetened chocolate
- 2 large avocados
- 2 tsp. vanilla extract
- 1 cup coconut milk
- ½ cup heavy whipping cream
- ½ cup unsweetened cocoa powder
- ½ cup powdered erythritol

Directions:

1. You are going to need to blend the avocado, coconut milk, cream, and vanilla extract in a blender until fully combined. The mixture should be smooth and lime green in color.

2. Add the powdered erythritol, liquid Stevia, and cocoa powder to the creamy mixture, and blend together until fully combined.

3. Break the unsweetened chocolate squares into chunky pieces and add to the coffee brown creamy mixture, and freeze together in a medium-large bowl for 8 hours.

4. Use the freeze and stir method to get that creamy ice cream texture and you are going to need to put the ice cream in a shallow dish container for this part.

5. Put the ice cream in the freezer for 30 minutes, then remove and stir the ice cream, and then put the ice cream back in the freezer for 30 minutes.

6. You should repeat the above-mentioned action for 3 hours, until the ice cream starts sticking and molding to the container.

7. Once the process is complete, you can serve and enjoy.

Berry Pops

Berry Pops are popsicles you can make with the use of blueberries and raspberries —two major keto-friendly fruits. This is an ideal dessert recipe that even your non-keto following family and friends will enjoy.

A few notes for this recipe:

- You will need popsicle molds and sticks.
- You can substitute the coconut cream with the whole cream.
- If you want to use strawberries instead of raspberries or blueberries, check the intake of macros first.

When you start freezing the molds, use the times as suggestions because some freezers—like mine—do not freeze liquids quickly enough, so allow for extra time if you have the same issue with your freezer.

The recipe below yields 6 Berry Pops.

Time: 5 hours

Serving Size: 1

Prep Time: 3 hours

Cook Time: 2 hours

Nutritional Facts/Info:

Calories: 146.33

Carbs: 5.26 grams

Fat: 13.07 grams

Protein: 1.14 grams

Ingredients:

- 1 ½ tsp. liquid Stevia
- 1 ½ cup canned coconut cream
- 1 cup frozen raspberries
- 1 cup frozen blueberries
- 1 cup water
- ½ tsp. vanilla extract

Directions:

1. You will need to use two small- to medium-sized pots to set to boil at medium-high temperature. In one pot, you will cook the raspberries, ½ cup of water, and ½ tsp. of liquid Stevia together. In the second pot, you will need to cook ½ cup of water, ½ tsp. of liquid Stevia, and blueberries.

2. Both of the raspberries and the blueberries mixtures should boil for 5 minutes before you can take them off the stove. Allow the mixtures to cool slightly—you do not want the heat to crack your glass blender if you transfer the too-hot liquid in the blender.

3. Blend the raspberry and blueberry separately until smooth and pour them out into separate bowls before allowing them to cool in the fridge.

4. Use a jug (this makes it easier for pouring) or a small bowl to mix together the coconut cream, ½ liquid Stevia, and vanilla extract.

Put the mixture in the fridge for later use.

5. Imagine a traffic light for the next part, well if the green light was red (raspberry mixture), the yellow light was white (coconut cream mixture), and the red light was blue (blueberry mixture). You would need to layer and fill your molds in the same way.

6. Scoop 3 tbsp. of raspberry mix into the molds and put the mold in the freezer for 1 hour.

7. Scoop 4 tbsp. of coconut mix into the same mold once the raspberry has set and put the mold in the freezer for 30 minutes.

8. Insert sticks into each mold; the coconut mix should be semi-set to properly hold the sticks, and put the mold back in the freezer for 1 hour.

9. The last 3 scoops to be placed into the mold is the blueberry mixture; after you have scooped the blueberry mix into the mold, place the mold back into the

freezer for a maximum of 2 hours.

10. And once the pops have set, you can enjoy your tasty summer-time fruity dessert.

Tomato Soup

Tomato Soup is exactly what you need on those cold winter nights when you just want to hug a bowl of warm soup to your chest.

The recipe below can make 4 bowls of Tomato Soup.

Time: 35 minutes

Serving Size: 1 bowl

Prep Time: 10 minutes

Cook Time: 25 minutes

Nutritional Facts/Info:

Calories: 301.5

Carbs: 8.75 grams

Fat: 25.79 grams

Protein: 9.29 grams

Ingredients:

- 1 x 6 oz. can of tomato paste
- 1 cup heavy whipping cream
- 1 tsp. oregano
- 1 tsp. garlic powder
- ½ tsp. kosher salt
- ¼ cup water
- ¾ cup shredded parmesan cheese

Directions:

1. First, you will need a medium-sized pot. Place this on the stove and set the plate to a low-medium heat.
2. Shortly after that, throw in the tomato paste and garlic and stir the ingredients together until they are smoothly combined.
3. Once the tomato paste and garlic are combined, add the cream to

the mix, which will lighten the color of the soup, and stir until the soup begins to simmer.

4. When the soup starts to bubble, you can add in the cheese, a teaspoon full at a time until the soup starts to thicken, at which point you can pour in ¼ cup of water and cook the soup for another 5 minutes.

5. You can serve immediately or reheat for later enjoyment.

Roasted Broccoli

Roasted Broccoli is an excellent side dish that could be paired with some fried cauliflower rice or another keto-friendly dinner meal. They are also so quick and easy to make, so you do not even have to wonder if they will be worth your time to pair with your meal.

This recipe makes a total of 6 servings, and the leftovers can be stored in a sealable container in the freezer and reheated for other meals, although they won't be as crunchy.

Time: 30 minutes

Serving Size: 1

Prep Time: 5 minutes

Cook Time: 25 minutes

Nutritional Facts/Info:

Calories: 138.17

Carbs: 5.24 grams

Fat: 10.77 grams

Protein: 4.83 grams

Ingredients:

- 3 tsp. garlic powder
- 2 tbsp. chopped fresh basil
- 1 ½ pound broccoli florets
- ⅓ cup Parmesan cheese
- ½ tsp. kosher salt
- ½ tsp. red chili flakes
- ½ lemon juice and zest

- ¼ cup olive oil

Directions:

1. Turn on the oven and set the temperature to 425 degrees Fahrenheit.
2. Use silicone baking pads to cover the bottom of your baking tray, lay the broccoli florets out on the tray, and drizzle the broccoli with olive oil, freshly chopped basil, garlic powder, kosher salt, red chili flakes, lemon zest (grated lemon skin), and lemon juice.
3. Shower the broccoli with Parmesan cheese and put the tray in the oven for 25 minutes before serving right out of the oven for your enjoyment.

Low-Carb Cauliflower Hash Browns

Low-Carb Cauliflower Hash Browns are a great breakfast dish on their own, but they can also be a wonderful breakfast side-dish. You could pair them with anything or, as is traditional, top them off with some sour cream or fried scallions.

These hash browns are crunchy, keto-friendly, and easy to throw together and make.

You should use a keto-friendly butter if you want to use butter, which you can drizzle over the hash browns when done, but in this recipe, we make use of olive oil for frying.

This recipe yields 4 servings you can store in the fridge in a sealable container.

Time: 25 minutes

Serving Size: 1

Prep Time: 10 minutes

Cook Time: 10 minutes

Nutritional Facts/Info:

Calories: 331

Carbs: 8.5 grams

Fat: 31.9 grams

Protein: 7.3 grams

Ingredients:

- 16 oz. of cauliflower
- 1 small onion
- 3 large eggs
- 1 tsp garlic salt
- Pinch of pepper
- 8 tbsp of olive oil

Directions:

1. Start by washing your vegetables and then proceed by breaking the cauliflower into florets and blending them in your food processor. They should resemble little grains of white fluffy rice.

2. Next, grate your onion and add it to the cauliflower before adding the mix to a medium-sized bowl. Add in the eggs, garlic salt, pepper, and any other seasoning of your choice, and mix together

before setting the mixture aside for 10 minutes.

3. During the 10 minutes that the mixture sets, you can start pouring olive oil into a medium heated frying pan.

4. Scoop out the hash brown size you want into the frying pan; do not turn the hash brown too early, rather wait until it is golden brown on one side or else it may crumble.

5. Each side of the hash brown should be fried for 3 to 4 minutes and you can add more oil to the frying pan if needed.

6. Finally, once the hash browns are cooked, you can enjoy them with your own choice of toppings.

Creamy Spinach

Creamy Spinach consists of spinach and a creamy Parmesan and cream cheese mixture, which is the essence of this delicious side meal.

The recipe below yields 3 servings and the leftovers can be stored in the fridge and reheated in the microwave for another meal.

Time: 20 minutes

Serving Size: 1

Prep Time: 5 minutes

Cook Time: 15 minutes

Nutritional Facts/Info:

Calories: 165

Carbs: 3.63 grams

Fat: 13.22 grams

Protein: 7.33 grams

Ingredients:

- ¼ tsp. onion powder
- 10 oz. frozen spinach
- 3 oz. cream cheese
- 3 tbsp. Parmesan cheese

- 2 tbsp sour cream
- ¼ tsp. garlic powder

Directions:

1. Take the spinach out of the freezer and allow the spinach to defrost at room temperature through the day.
2. Cook the spinach in a saucepan on a medium heat until the excess water from the spinach has dried out.
3. Sprinkle the spinach with garlic powder, onion powder, and any other seasoning of your choice.
4. Now, stir in the cream cheese and allow the cream cheese to melt into the spinach before adding the sour cream into the spinach, and then melting the Parmesan into the spinach.
5. Stir the creamed spinach for another 2 minutes before serving as a side dish.

The Bottom Line

You have got options!

We hope you have learned for the last two chapters. You have tons of food options and ideas to try out; however, you must be willing and ready to get into the kitchen and learn to prepare your own meals.

The best way to partake in a vegetarian ketogenic diet is learning to prepare your own foods, which should also encourage you to come up with new tasty recipes that could expand the options we have as vegetarians.

However, there are wonderful recipes that are part of this chapter that you can try out. You could alter them to meet your needs; they are really tasty and worthwhile.

But don't think there are just six recipes for you! The next couple of chapters are jammed-packed with tasty recipes for you to try out.

Chapter 5: Vegetarian Keto Diet Breakfast Ideas

Blueberry Pancakes

Blueberry Pancakes are low in carbohydrates and quite an excellent and an enjoyable breakfast. The golden pancakes are light and fluffy and not too sweet. You can pair the pancakes with a keto-friendly syrup, but these pancakes are pretty tasty on their own.

What you are going to need to make these pancakes is a large mixing bowl, an electric mixer, a ladle, a spatula, measuring cups and spoons, and lastly, your trusted pancake-making pan, which is just my way of referring to a non-stick pan. When it comes to short-term storing of the pancakes, you can place the pancakes in a sealable container and store them in your fridge, but for long-term storage, it is better to keep them in your freezer and defrost them in the microwave.

The recipe yields 4 Blueberry Pancakes.

Time: 12 minutes

Serving Size: 1

Prep Time: 10 minutes

Cook Time: 2 to 3 minutes on each side or until golden brown.

Nutritional Facts/Info:

Calories: 389.25

Carbs: 7.23 grams

Fat: 33.26 grams

Protein: 19.05 grams

Ingredients:

- 3 large eggs
- 1 cup almond flour
- 1 tsp. baking powder
- ½ tsp. vanilla extract
- ½ cup golden flaxseed meal
- ¼ cup unsweetened vanilla almond milk
- ¾ cup ricotta cream
- ¼ tsp. salt
- ½ tsp. Stevia powder
- ¼ cup blueberries

Directions:

1. Set the above-mentioned ingredients out on the kitchen counter, take out your measuring cups and spoon, and start by whisking the three eggs until frothy in your mixing bowl.
2. Pour vanilla extract, ricotta cream, and the almond milk to the eggs and gently mix the ingredients together with an electric whisk.

3. Proceed by adding Stevia, almond flour, and baking powder into the bowl, gently whisk the ingredients together, then add in the flaxseed meal and salt, and whisk until smooth.
4. Set the mixture aside.
5. Now, place the pan on the stove and set the temperature to a medium heat, and while you wait, cut your berries in half.
6. Check the heat of the pan by sprinkling some water in it, and if the water sizzles, then you can add a small amount of butter to grease the pan.
7. Use a ladle to pour the pancake mixture into the hot pan, place 6 halved berries on the pancake, and use a spatula to flip the pancakes when the edges begin to brown.
8. Repeat the above process to make three other pancakes.
9. Once done, place the yellow-golden pancakes on a plate, and

top them off with a keto-friendly topping of your choice.

Low-Carb Brownie Muffins

Low-Carb Brownie Muffins are a yummy breakfast to make and have on-the-go, and with a yield of 4 tasty and chewy muffins, you can already save the other two for the next day's breakfast, thus saving time and money.

What you are going to need to make this high fiber breakfast muffin is a large mixing bowl, an electric mixer, measuring cups and spoons, and your keto-friendly ingredients.

You can store any remaining muffins in a sealable container and enjoy these later.

Time: 25 minutes

Serving Size: 1 muffin

Prep Time: 10 minutes

Cook Time: 15 minutes

Nutritional Facts/Info:

Calories: 289.5

Carbs: 6.55 grams

Fat: 21.14 grams

Protein: 10.47 grams

Ingredients:

- 2 tbsp. coconut oil
- 1 cup golden flaxseed meal
- 1 tbsp. cinnamon
- 1 large egg
- 1 tsp. vanilla extract
- 1 tsp. apple cider vinegar
- ¼ cup cocoa powder
- ½ tbsp. baking powder
- ½ tsp. salt
- ¼ cup sugar-free caramel syrup
- ½ cup pumpkin purée
- ¼ cup slivered almonds

Directions:

1. Start by turning the oven on and setting the temperature to 350 degrees Fahrenheit.

2. Break the egg into the large mixing bowl, add in the coconut oil and caramel syrup, and blend using the electric mixer. The mixture will be yellow in color and have a sticky texture.

3. Now pour in the vanilla extract, apple cider vinegar, and pumpkin purée and whisk together with the mixer. The mixture should still be yellow but more watery in texture.

4. Mix in the cocoa powder, flaxseed, cinnamon, slivered almonds, and salt to the yellow mixture, and combine until the mixture is brown and grain-like in texture.

5. Spray your muffin pan with non-stick baking spray or grease four muffin molds with coconut oil. Scoop the mixture into the 4

molds and bake the muffins for 12 to 15 minutes.

6. Allow the muffins to cool before removing them from the molds and enjoying right away.

Veggie Scramble

Veggie Scramble is the crunchy and fluffy egged morning breakfast. Our recipe is bursting with colors and flavors and really fantastic spices.

You can use other keto-friendly vegetables and spices for this scramble. For example, you can substitute the eggs with more thinly sliced baby mushrooms.

This recipe makes 2 dishes.

Time: 25 minutes

Serving Size: 1

Prep Time: 15 minutes

Cook Time: 10 minutes

Nutritional Facts/Info:

Calories: 311

Carbs: 4.9 grams

Fat: 24.5 grams

Protein: 14.2 grams

Ingredients:

- ¼ cup olive oil
- ¼ red onions
- ½ tsp. salt
- ½ tsp. turmeric powder
- 1 cup chopped spinach
- 1 tbsp. coconut milk
- 1 tsp. cayenne pepper
- 1 tsp. garlic powder
- 4 baby mushrooms
- 4 eggs
- 4 mini bell peppers

Directions:

1. Start by placing a pan on the stove at a low-medium heat and pour olive oil in the pan.
2. Cut the baby mushrooms into slices, chop the spinach, red onions, and bell peppers, and place the ingredients in the pan to fry until onions or peppers start to brown around the edges.
3. Use a small-medium bowl to beat the eggs until foam starts to form, whisk in the coconut milk and salt, and add the mixture to the pan and scramble the ingredients together until the eggs are cooked to your liking.
4. Add the turmeric, cayenne pepper, and garlic powder to the mix, cook for 5 minutes and scramble with a fork, and dish it out right away and serve.

Keto Breakfast Granola

Keto Breakfast Granola is the crunchy morning breakfast you will enjoy with that full-fat and no-sugar Greek yogurt. There will also be enough left over from this recipe to have for your breakfast for at least a week and a half to two weeks.

Talking about leftovers, you can store the granola in the fridge to ensure it remains crispy and crunchy. You can also swap in the nuts for your own choice of nuts but ensure you don't overindulge.

The recipe below yields 15 Keto Breakfast Granola servings.

Time: 25 minutes

Serving Size: ½ cup

Prep Time: 5 minutes

Cook Time: 35 minutes

Nutritional Facts/Info:

Calories: 169

Carbs: 5 grams

Fat: 16 grams

Protein: 4 grams

Ingredients:

- 5 tablespoon coconut oil
- 3 cups coconut flakes
- 1 cup raw macadamia nuts
- ½ cup raw almonds
- ¼ walnuts
- ¼ pumpkin seeds
- 2 tsp. chia seed
- 1 tsp. cinnamon powder

Directions:

1. Turn the oven on to 250 degrees Fahrenheit.
2. You can chop your almonds, macadamia, and walnuts, or you can blend them together in your food processor.
3. Pour the nuts into a bowl and mix in the pumpkin and chia seeds, cinnamon powder, coconut flakes, and coconut oil together until nicely combined.
4. Proceed with lining a baking tray

with wax paper and then spread the nuts and seeds out on the tray.

5. Place the tray in the oven for 35 minutes and rotate the nuts halfway through.

6. Remove the tray from the oven and cool before serving with keto-friendly yogurt or toppings of your choice.

Mixed Berry Smoothie

This keto mixed berry smoothie is a truly *sweet* way to start your morning.

A mixed berry smoothie does not seem like the greatest idea in the world when you are on the keto diet; however, the secret is to choose the correct berries. Strawberries and raspberries are keto-friendly, but you can throw in some blackberries for extra flavor.

Nevertheless, to thicken the smoothie, you could throw in ice cubes or avocados. And you can add some chia seeds in there too for extra thickness and more nutrient benefits.

Time: 5 minutes

Serving Size: cup

Prep Time: 5 minutes

Nutritional Facts/Info:

Calories: 388

Carbs: 13.1 grams

Fat: 38.3 grams

Protein: 3.9 grams

Ingredients:

- 3 cubes of ice
- ¼ cup of mixed berries (raspberry, strawberry, and blackberry)
- ½ tsp erythritol (optional)
- ⅔ cup of coconut milk

Directions:

1. Blend ice cubes for 10 seconds in the blender or until crushed.
2. Now add in the raspberries, strawberries, blackberries, erythritol, and coconut milk into the blender and combine until smooth and pink.
3. Serve chilled, and you can sprinkle some chia seeds on top.

Low-Carb Oatmeal

Low-Carb Oatmeal can cure that oatmeal craving that you may have.

This is a quick and easy to make breakfast meal that is high in protein, moderate in fat, and low in carbs, so it is a great after-workout breakfast meal and totally worth your time.

You could either use a keto-friendly milk of your choice or stick to water for this recipe. The recipe below serves one person, but if you wish to make extra, then simply double the ingredients by the amount of people you want to serve.

Furthermore, this meal is higher in carbs, so ensure you stay within your macro counts with regard to your meals the rest of the day.

Time: 8 minutes

Serving Size: 1 bowl

Prep Time: 1 minute

Cook Time: 5 minutes

Nutritional Facts/Info:

Calories: 274

Carbs: 21.7 grams

Fat: 18.4 grams

Protein: 9.5 grams

Ingredients:

- ½ cup of coconut milk

- 3 tbsp of almond meal
- 1 tbsp of coconut flour
- 1 tsp of chia seeds
- ½ of cinnamon

Directions:

1. Pour the coconut milk into a small pot, set the temperature on the stove to a medium heat, and allow the milk to simmer.
2. Stir in the almond meal, coconut flour, chia seeds, Stevia, and cinnamon.
3. Allow the oatmeal to boil for 1 minute at the same heat before dishing out into a breakfast bowl.

Chapter 6: Vegetarian Keto Diet Lunch Ideas

Collard Green Veggie Wraps

Collard Green Veggie Wraps are a mouthwatering lunch and also a dinner option. They are bursting in veggie colors, crunchy and scrumptious, and the tzatziki sauce makes you wish every meal tasted this good.

Imagine sushi but the fish is collard green leaves, and the stuffing is cucumber, red bell pepper, purple onion, Kalamata olives, feta cheese, and cherry tomatoes.

There is so much flavor in this one lunch meal for you to enjoy! You can prepare the wraps the night before and store it in a sealable container before placing the container in the fridge for later use.

With the recipe below, you can make 4 servings of Collard Green Veggie Wraps.

Time: 25 minutes

Serving Size: 1 wrap

Prep Time: 25 minutes

Cook Time: N/A

Nutritional Facts/Info:

Calories: 165.34 grams

Carbs: 7.36 grams

Fat: 11.25 grams

Protein: 6.98 grams

Ingredients:

- 2.5 oz. cucumber
- 2 tbsp. olive oil
- 2 tbsp. minced fresh dill
- 1 cup full-fat plain Greek yogurt
- 1 tsp. garlic powder
- 1 tbsp. white vinegar
- 8 Kalamata olives
- 4 large collard green leaves
- 4 cherry tomatoes
- 1 medium cucumber
- ½ medium red bell pepper
- ½ cup purple onion
- ½ block feta

Directions:

1. You will begin by making the tzatziki sauce, which you should store in the fridge for later use, and you are going to need a small- to medium-sized bowl for this.

2. Grate the cucumber on a cutting board first to ensure the excess water from the cucumber is not mixed into the tzatziki.

3. Transfer the cucumber into the bowl, then add in the olive oil,

minced fresh dill, full-fat plain Greek yogurt, garlic powder, and white vinegar. Stir the ingredients together until they resemble a white paste.

4. And now for the wrap, you will need to wash all the ingredients for the wrap.

5. Cut the Kalamata olives and cherry tomatoes in half.

6. Dice the purple onion and cut the feta cheese into one-inch thick strips.

7. Cut the cucumber and red bell pepper into strips (like fries).

8. Cut the stems off the collard green leaves and thickly 'butter' each leaf with tzatziki sauce.

9. Proceed with topping the leaves with the cucumber slices, then the pepper, onion, olives, feta, and the tomatoes in the center of the wrap. Fold the wraps like a burrito (fold the sides and then fold the middle).

10. Cut the wraps in half and use the rest of the sauce on top of your wraps for extra deliciousness.

Red Pepper Spinach Salad

Red Pepper Spinach Salad is a great light lunch salad to have on those days where you need to keep your calorie count down, so you can maybe enjoy some keto chocolate ice cream for dessert without the guilt.

This is a quick and easy meal to make and to enjoy on those really busy days.

The recipe below yields 2 servings of Red Pepper Spinach Salad.

Time: 10 minutes

Serving Size: 1 bowl

Prep Time: 10 minutes

Cook Time: N/A

Nutritional Facts/Info:

Calories: 212.68

Carbs: 5.01 grams

Fat: 19.49 grams

Protein: 6.5 grams

Ingredients:

- 6 cups spinach
- 3 tbsp. Parmesan cheese
- 1 tsp. red pepper flakes
- ¼ cup ranch dressing

Directions:

1. Throw together the spinach and the ranch dressing in a bowl until nicely combined.
2. Once the spinach and ranch are combined, then mix in the Parmesan cheese and sprinkle the mix with red pepper flakes.
3. Serve and enjoy.

Keto Club Salad

Keto Club Salad is so worth to diet for!

Imagine a bowl filled to the rim with red, yellow, green, and white. This is a truly filling lunch meal with a satisfying crunch.

The recipe below should provide you with 3 servings, and you can store any leftovers by sealing them in a container and putting the container in your fridge.

Time: 35 minutes

Serving Size: 1 bowl

Prep Time: 15 minutes

Cook Time: 20 minutes

Nutritional Facts/Info:

Calories: 329.67

Carbs: 4.83 grams

Fat: 26.32 grams

Protein: 16.82 grams

Ingredients:

- 4 oz. cheddar cheese
- 3 large eggs
- 3 cups iceberg lettuce
- 2 tbsp. sour cream
- 2 tbsp. mayonnaise
- 1 tsp. dried parsley
- 1 ½ tbsp. milk
- 1 cup cucumber
- 1 tbsp. Dijon mustard
- ½ tsp. garlic powder
- ½ tsp onion powder
- ½ cup cherry tomatoes

Directions:

1. Start by getting out all the above-mentioned ingredients, a medium-sized bowl, a cutting board, and a small-medium pot.
2. You should lay everything you need on a clean kitchen counter top and ensure you thoroughly wash your vegetables.
3. Firstly, pour some water into the pot, put the pot on medium heat on the stove, put the eggs in the water, cover the pot, and allow the eggs to harden in the water.

The suggested time is about 9 minutes for a medium-sized egg, 12 minutes for a large egg, and longer for bigger eggs.

4. While the eggs are boiling, start cutting your vegetables on the cutting board. Start by tearing the iceberg lettuce to pieces, cut the cheddar cheese into cubes, cut your cherry tomatoes in half, and dice your cucumber.

5. Place every ingredient in the bowl once you are done cutting, tearing, and dicing them.

6. The eggs should be boiled at this point, so remove the pot from the plate, and pour cold water from the tap into the pot so the eggs cool down much quicker and they stop cooking.

7. While you wait on the eggs to cool, make the dressing by stirring together, in a small bowl, the sour cream, mayonnaise, milk, garlic powder, onion powder, and dried parsley. The dressing should not be too

watery. Store in the fridge for later use.

8. And now you can peel the eggs, cut them in half, and place them in the bowl with the rest of the salad.

9. Stir your salad, mixing the colors together, squirt some Dijon mustard in the center of the salad, and coat the salad in the dressing.

10. Cover the leftovers and store in the refrigerator.

Grilled Cheese Zucchini

Grilled Cheese Zucchini is not exactly as weird as it sounds; the zucchini is the sandwich and man, does the zucchini taste like the best darn keto-friendly sandwich ever. You are seriously going to enjoy this crispy and crunchy filling 'sandwich.'

What you are going to need is a spatula, frying pan, cutting board, and all the ingredients listed below.

This recipe makes 3 servings, so you can make one 'sandwich' to enjoy now and store the rest away for another day in the week, therefore, saving you time and money.

Time: 25 minutes

Serving Size: 1 'sandwich'

Prep Time: 10 minutes

Cook Time: 15 minutes

Nutritional Facts/Info:

Calories: 300

Carbs: 4 grams

Fat: 14 grams

Protein: 20 grams

Ingredients:

- 2 cup grated zucchini
- 2 cup shredded cheddar

- 2 green onions
- 1 large egg
- ½ cup freshly grated Parmesan
- ¼ cup cornstarch
- ½ tsp. basil powder
- A pinch of salt and pepper
- Olive oil

Directions:

1. Wash your zucchini before grating 2 cups worth of zucchini onto your cutting board, then grate the Parmesan cheese into a mixing bowl, and add the zucchini to the same mixing bowl.

2. Whisk your egg in a small bowl with salt, pepper, and basil; then add this mix into the mixing bowl of zucchini and Parmesan.

3. Cut your onion into thin slices and add the onion slices and cornstarch to the mixing bowl before mixing the ingredients together. The mixture should resemble a white batter.

4. Now, take your frying pan, put it on the stove, set the temperature

on the plate to a medium heat, and pour enough olive oil to cover the pan.

5. Use a spoon and flatten out 4 tablespoons of the batter onto the pan, and form these into a square.

6. Fry the zucchini on both sides until golden, and then move the zucchini to a plate, fry another slice, and repeat the action until you have the amount of Grilled Cheese Zucchini 'slices' that you want.

7. Place a cooked zucchini back on the pan, spread cheddar or your cheese of choice onto the zucchini, and place another cooked zucchini on top. Wait for the cheese to melt before flipping over, and do this for all your other zucchini 'slices' and fry each for a 1 or 2 minutes.

8. Place the 'sandwich' on a plate, cut in two, and enjoy.

Asparagus Fries

Asparagus Fries is a great snack, an equally amazing side dish, and easy lunch time meal. The majority of fat (42.57 grams) in this recipe comes from the 3 tbsp of mayonnaise. The 10 medium asparagus spears contain 6.21 grams of carbs and 3.4 grams of fiber, and the ½ cup of shredded Parmesan cheese provides the most protein at 15.14 grams.

Ensure your mayonnaise is keto-friendly, but if you don't, you can make homemade mayonnaise with the provided ingredients below.

The recipe makes a total of 2 servings, and the homemade mayonnaise amounts to 1 ¼ cups worth of mayonnaise.

Time: 30 minutes

Serving Size: 1

Prep Time: 20 minutes

Cook Time: 10 minutes

Nutritional Facts/Info:

Calories: 453.65

Carbs: 5.51 grams

Fat: 33.43 grams

Protein: 19.14 grams

Ingredients: Asparagus Fries

- 10 medium asparagus spears
- 3 tbsp. mayonnaise
- 2 large eggs
- 2 tbsp. chopped parsley
- 1 tbsp. roasted and chopped red pepper
- ½ cup shredded Parmesan cheese
- ½ tsp. garlic powder
- ½ tsp. smoked paprika
- ¼ cup almond flour

Ingredients: Mayonnaise

- 3 drops liquid Stevia

- 2 large egg yolks
- 1 large egg
- 1 tsp. Dijon mustard
- ½ cup melted coconut oil
- ¾ cup olive oil
- A pinch of salt
- A pinch of smoked paprika

Directions:

1. Preheat the oven to 425 degrees Fahrenheit.
2. Unless you have a keto-friendly mayonnaise, start by making your mayonnaise: soften the coconut oil in the microwave, which should take 20 to 60 seconds. Shortly after that, pour and mix the olive oil in a small-medium bowl.
3. Pour egg yolks, liquid Stevia, egg, Dijon mustard, salt, and smoked paprika into your blender, blend the ingredients, and add the oil in little by little (drops) until the mayonnaise *emulsifies*, and only after that can you start adding the

oil more frequently between pulses.

4. Transfer the mayo to a sealable container and you can keep it in the fridge. The mayo will last for a maximum of 3 weeks. If you want the mayo to last for much longer, you will need to add 1 tbsp. of whey to the mix and allow they mayo to set for roughly 8 hours before you can refrigerate it.

5. You are going to need to use a small-medium container to combine the chopped roasted red pepper and mayonnaise together. Allow the mayo pepper mix to chill in the refrigerator.

6. And now take the Parmesan cheese, parsley, and garlic powder and place these ingredients in your blender, and mix until smooth. Add the ¼ cup of almond flour, and mix until the mixture resembles bread crumbs.

7. Pour the mixture onto a kitchen tray and season the mixture with the smoked paprika.

8. Whisk the eggs in a medium-sized container (you will need to be able to coat the asparagus in this bowl, so ensure the container is large enough for this process) until the eggs start to foam.

9. Now coat the asparagus in the egg mix, then you have to hold the asparagus over the 'bread crumb' mixture and sprinkle the mixture over the asparagus.

10. Transfer every piece of asparagus straight to the baking tray after coating them in the 'bread crumb' mixture, and once all the asparagus has been coated, pour any leftover mixture over the asparagus in the tray.

11. Place the tray in the oven and bake for 10 minutes or until the 'bread crumbs' begin to brown.

12. After taking the asparagus out of the oven, you can begin consuming your crispy warm fries

with your homemade red pepper aioli.

Avocado Taco

Avocado Taco is an amazing and flavorful lunch or even a dinner time dish, filled with healthy good fats, and a hearty combo of nuts and vegetables.

And what you are going to need for this is a grinder, a frying pan, as well as the yummy keto-friendly ingredients listed below.

There should be enough taco filling for two avocados, so you can save the leftover taco filling in a sealable bag and store in your freezer for lunch during the week or to have the same dinner later in the evening.

Time: 20 minutes

Serving Size: ½ avocado

Prep Time: 10 minutes

Cook Time: 10 minutes

Nutritional Facts/Info:

Calories: 454

Carbs: 6.5 grams

Fat: 40 grams

Protein: 16 grams

Ingredients:

- 1 cup raw walnuts
- 1 tbsp. hulled hemp seeds
- 1 tsp. cumin
- 1 tsp. garlic powder
- 1 tsp. salt
- ½ cup chopped onion
- ½ medium avocado
- 3 tbsp. shredded cheddar cheese
- 2 tsp. adobo sauce
- 4 tsp. smoked paprika
- 4 tbsp. avocado oil
- 7 oz. cauliflower

Directions:

1. Get out all the above-mentioned ingredients and start by cutting your onion into thin slices and placing them in the grinder with cauliflower florets, raw walnuts, hemp seeds, cumin, garlic powder, and lastly, the salt or a seasoning of your choice.

2. Place a large pan on the stove and set it to a low temperature, and add in 2 tbsp. of avocado oil.

3. Grind the ingredients together until the mixture you see in your grinder resembles tiny bread crumbs. Note: if your pan isn't large enough to fit in the mixture, then divide the mixture in two.

4. Set the temperature on the pan to a medium heat and add in the mixture, use a spatula or wooden spoon for stirring, and cook 2 to 4 minutes before adding 2 tbsp. adobo sauce (if you are only cooking half, then use 1 tbsp. of adobo sauce).

5. Cook for 5 more minutes; the taco filling should be brown in color

and look like minced meat. Add in the 2 tbsp. of cheddar cheese (1 tbsp. if cooking in halves).

6. Cut your avocado in 2 and remove the seed.

7. Dig out enough space in your avocado for the taco filling, stuff the avocado with the taco filling you just made, and top the filling with 1 tbsp. of cheddar and the previously dug out avocado.

Mushroom & Avocado Salad

Mushroom & Avocado Salad is another amazing lunch time meal, and the buttered mushrooms really ties the entire meal together.

You are seriously going to enjoy this flexible meal that allows for all sorts of alterations and add-ins. What you are going to need to make this dish is a pan, spatula, and the ingredients you can find in the list below.

The recipe below makes one bowl of Mushroom & Avocado Salad.

Time: 15 minutes

Serving Size: 1

Prep Time: 5 minutes

Cook Time: 10 minutes

Nutritional Facts/Info:

Calories: 617

Carbs: 7 grams

Fat: 55. 7 grams

Protein: 17.5 grams

Ingredients:

- 1 avocado
- 1 oz. goat cheese
- 1 tbsp. balsamic vinegar
- 1 tbsp. butter
- 1 tbsp. olive oil

- 2 oz. cremini mushrooms
- 4 oz. spring mix
- Salt and pepper

Directions:

1. Start by gathering all the ingredients and crumbling your goat cheese, cutting the avocado into small cubed pieces, and cutting the mushrooms into slices.

2. Now, place your pan on the stove and set the temperature to a medium heat.

3. While you wait for the pan to warm up, take a bowl and pour in the spring mix, crumbled cheese, and cubed avocados.

4. Place 1 tbsp. of butter in the pan and add the mushroom in. Once the butter has melted, and sprinkle with salt and pepper. Allow the mushrooms to cook until golden brown and add them to the salad.

5. Use a small bowl to combine 1 tbsp. of olive oil and 1 tbsp. of balsamic vinegar.
6. Coat the salad with the olive oil balsamic vinegar combo, mix the salad together, and you can dig into a delicious lunch time salad.

Chapter 7: Vegetarian Keto Diet Dinner Ideas

Keto Broccoli Salad

Keto Broccoli Salad is a great dinner option that allows you to get all your healthy and keto-friendly veggies in for the day.

There are so many fun flavors and colors in this one dish that it is darn near inspiring. Essentially, this is the meal that could make you really content with eating healthy.

You can opt to cook the broccoli in boiling water for five minutes on a medium heat or eat the broccoli raw. You could also use thinly chopped almonds instead of pumpkin seeds.

The recipe yields 8 servings.

Time: 25 minutes

Serving Size: 1

Prep Time: 25 minutes

Cook Time: N/A

Nutritional Facts/Info:

Calories: 357.13

Carbs: 3.95 grams

Fat: 32.01 grams

Protein: 12.11 grams

Ingredients:

- ½ cup pumpkin seeds
- ½ medium red onion
- ¾ cup mayonnaise
- 1 large avocado
- 3 cups broccoli florets
- 3 tbsp. apple cider vinegar

- 4 oz. cheddar cheese
- 5 tablespoon erythritol
- Salt and pepper

Directions:

1. In a small container, mix together the mayonnaise, erythritol, and the apple cider vinegar to make the dressing for the salad.
2. Set the dressing aside and wash your vegetables, and on a cutting board, cut the broccoli into bite-size pieces and place the pieces in a medium-large sized bowl.
3. Dice half of a red onion and add it to the bowl.
4. Cut your cheddar into cubes and add to the bowl.
5. Then cut your avocado into slices, then cut the slices in three, and add them to the mix.
6. Pour the dressing over the bowl and combine the vegetables.
7. Serve and enjoy.

Zucchini Skins

Zucchini Skins can be used for a quick and easy to make keto dinner, or it can even be made and served as an appetizer.

You may substitute the squash for another low carb keto-friendly squash.

Three zucchini is worth 11.01 grams of carbs and 3.5 grams of fiber, the 2 oz. of cheddar is worth 18.89 grams of fat, and 2 oz. of pepper jack cheese contains 13.88 grams of protein.

When it comes to storing the zucchini skins, you can place them in a sealable container in the fridge and use the microwave to reheat them prior to serving.

The recipe yields 6 servings worth of zucchini skins.

Time: 35 minutes

Serving Size: 6

Prep Time: 15 minutes

Cook Time: 20 minutes

Nutritional Facts/Info:

Calories: 108.5

Carbs: 2.82 grams

Fat: 8.25 grams

Protein: 5.76 grams

Ingredients:

- 3 small Zucchini
- 3 whole diced baby mushrooms
- 3 tbsp. sour cream
- 2 tsp. smoked paprika
- 2 oz. shredded cheddar cheese
- 2 oz. shredded Pepper Jack cheese
- 2 tbsp. chopped chives
- 1 tsp. olive oil
- 1 tbsp. Worcestershire sauce
- 1 ½ tsp salt

Directions:

1. Start by cutting the squashes right down the middle into six even halves; imagine them as little boats, and carve the seeds out of the zucchini with a spoon before sprinkling the slices with 1 tsp. of salt.

2. Next, you need to turn on your oven and set the temperature to 375 degrees Fahrenheit.

3. Use a small-medium container to prepare the diced mushrooms by dressing the mushrooms with the oil, smoked paprika, Worcestershire sauce, and ½ tsp. of salt.

4. On a baking tray, lay out the zucchini and mushrooms, place the tray in the oven, and allow it to cook until lightly browned.

5. Once you have taken the tray out of the oven, you can layer the zucchini with mushrooms, jack cheese, and the cheddar cheese.

6. Place the tray back in the oven and take the tray out of the oven once the cheeses begin to melt,

and enjoy the meal with some sour cream sprinkled with chopped chives.

Tofu & Bok Choy

Crispy Tofu & Bok Choy Salad is a tasty and crispy lunch time meal with a wonderful salad dressing. The majority of the fat (40.42 grams) in this recipe comes from the 3 tbsp. of coconut oil; 9 ounces of bok choy is worth 5.56 grams of carbs and 2.5 grams of fiber. The 3 tbsp. of soy sauce contain 3.91 grams of protein.

Some tips or alternatives for this recipe:

- You can substitute the monk fruit extract with Stevia.
- Remember to use a keto-friendly peanut butter.
- Also, you will need to dry out your tofu, which will take about 6 hours. Try drying the tofu the day

before, then marinate the tofu through the night. In the morning, you can place the tofu in the oven to bake and put the recipes together for your lunch. Store the leftovers in a sealable container and store away in your fridge. However, you can only store the crispy tofu for 3 days. When it comes to reheating the crispy tofu, you can use the microwave, but the tofu will not retain its crispiness. Therefore, we suggest using the oven and reheat the tofu at a temperature of 375 degrees Fahrenheit.

- The bok choy salad can be refrigerated for roughly five days. Store the leftover tofu, bok choy, and sauce separately, which will make it easier to reheat the tofu in the oven.

This recipe makes 3 servings.

Time: 8 hours 35 minutes

Serving Size: 1 bowl

Prep Time: 8 hours

Cook Time: 35 minutes

Nutritional Facts/Info:

Calories: 398.59

Carbs: 6.68 grams

Fat: 30.43 grams

Protein: 24.11 grams

Ingredients: Oven Baked Tofu

- 15 oz. extra firm tofu
- 2 teaspoons minced garlic
- ½ a lemon
- 1 tbsp. soy sauce
- 1 tbsp. sesame oil
- 1 tbsp. water
- 2 tsp. garlic powder
- 1 tbsp. rice wine vinegar

Ingredients: Bok Choy Salad

- 9 oz. ok choy
- 7 drops liquid monk fruit extract
- 3 tbsp. coconut oil
- 2 tbsp. chopped cilantro

- 2 tbsp. soy sauce
- 1 tbsp. sambal oelek
- 1 stalk green onion
- 1 tbsp. peanut butter
- ½ a lime

Directions:

1. Dry out your tofu with the assistance of two clean kitchen towels. First, lay the kitchen towel on a plate or kitchen tray, lay the tofu on the towel, put the second towel on top of the tofu, and then lay some heavy books — that you will not need for the next 6-hour processes—on top of the towel.

2. Once the tofu has been dried out with the use of towels, you need to fry-dry the tofu: cut the tofu into even slices, lay the slices out on a non-stick pan (no oil), and fry until the tofu is light brown in color. Cut the tofu into evenly sized squares.

3. Use a medium-sized container for the flavoring: mix together the

soy sauce, sesame oil, water, garlic, vinegar, and lemon juice.

4. In a sealable plastic bag, toss the tofu squares and the flavoring you just made together, and allow the flavors to soak in for 2 hours.

5. Once the tofu has marinated in the flavoring for the allotted time, proceed by preheating the oven at a temperature of 350 degrees Fahrenheit.

6. Line your baking tray with wax paper, lay the tofu on the tray, and bake in the oven for a maximum of 35 minutes or until the tofu is golden brown in color.

7. While the tofu is in the oven, cut the bok choy into small slices.

8. Continue by stirring together the chopped green onion and cilantro, coconut oil, soy sauce, sambal oelek, peanut butter, lime juice, and monk fruit extract in a small-medium bowl to make the salad dressing.

9. Once you remove the tofu from the oven, you can make your

Crispy Tofu & Bok Choy Salad by combining the tofu, bok choy, and sauce together.

10. Now get your chopsticks and enjoy.

Grilled Eggplant

Grilled Eggplant is a dinner dish with an amazing tasty sauce that really brings some true flavor to the grilled eggplant.

You are going to need a grill for this meal. Although the grilled eggplant is best served when warm, you can still store it in foil and refrigerate for serving the next day.

Our recipe only serves two but you can double the amount of eggplant to make extra and share with your non-vegetarian friends or family members. We are sure they will especially enjoy the tahini dressing.

Time: 30 minutes

Serving Size: 1

Prep Time: 20 minutes

Cook Time: 10 minutes

Nutritional Facts/Info:

Calories: 298

Carbs: 36.1 grams

Fat: 15.6 grams

Protein: 11.8 grams

Ingredients:

- 1 large eggplant
- 3 tbsp lemon juice
- 2 tbsp parsley
- ½ olive oil
- 1 tsp dried oregano
- ¼ tsp red pepper flakes
- A pinch of sea salt
- A pinch of black pepper
- ⅓ cup of tahini
- 2 tbsp water
- 1 tbsp garlic

Directions:

1. Use a medium-sized bowl to mix together tahini, lemon juice, water, and garlic, to make the tahini dressing, and then cover the bowl before putting it aside.
2. Use a medium-high heat for the grill. While the grill heats up, you can mix together the oil, oregano, and red pepper flakes in a small bowl.
3. Slice the eggplant into ¼--inch slices and lather the slices with the oil-oregano-pepper-flakes mix, and then place the slices on the grill.
4. Cook the slices for 3 minutes on each side or until golden yellow.
5. Lastly, drizzle the tahini dressing over the eggplant and enjoy.

Caprese Salad

Caprese Salad is a real summer time salad and a tasty Italian dish.

The is filled with the juices from grape tomatoes, the softness of mozzarella, and the healthy fats of avocado. What you are going to need for this meal is a serving bowl, a spoon, and the ingredients of course.

Time: 20 minutes

Serving Size: 1

Prep Time: 10 minutes

Cook Time: 10 minutes

Nutritional Facts/Info:

Calories: 284

Carbs: 8 grams

Fat: 26 grams

Protein: 6 grams

Ingredients:

- 1 cup balsamic vinegar
- ¼ cup extra virgin olive oil

- ¼ tsp. garlic powder
- ¼ tsp. sea salt
- ⅛ tsp. black pepper
- 2 cup grape tomatoes
- 1 cup mozzarella balls
- 1 medium avocado
- ⅓ cup fresh basil

Directions:

1. Start with cutting the grape tomatoes in half, dice the avocado, and chop the basil.
2. Put the tomatoes, avocado, and basil in a medium-sized bowl, and in another bowl, mix together the balsamic vinegar, olive oil, garlic powder, sea salt, and black pepper.
3. Add the balsamic olive oil mix to the bowl of tomatoes, avocado, basil and mix these together to ensure the salad is properly dressed.
4. Serve in a bowl and save any leftovers for later.

Broccoli Creamy Casserole

Broccoli Creamy Casserole is an enjoyable dinner time dish with keto-friendly vegetables, like cauliflower and broccoli, to create lovely colors and tasty flavors. As you go through the recipe, you may notice that the minced 'meat' is the same as the taco filing in the lunch chapter for the Avocado Taco recipe. Well, it is a great tasty mix that works as our minced 'meat' for his broccoli creamy casserole.

You can cook your broccoli first before putting it in the oven, but cook your broccoli in such a way that the crunchiness won't be lost unless it is something that doesn't matter to you.

The recipe below yields 8 servings.

Time: 1 hour 10 minutes

Serving Size: ⅛ Casserole

Prep Time: 10 minutes

Cook Time: 60 minutes

Nutritional Facts/Info:

Calories: 441

Carbs: 16.18 grams

Fat: 31.3 grams

Protein: 20.2 grams

Ingredients: Minced 'Meat'

- 1 cup raw walnuts
- 1 tbsp. hulled hemp seeds
- 1 tbsp. cheddar cheese
- 1 tsp. adobo sauce
- 1 tsp. garlic powder
- 1 tsp. onion powder
- 1 tsp. salt
- 2 tbsp. avocado oil
- 2 tsp. smoked paprika
- 4 oz. cauliflower

Ingredients: Broccoli Creamy Casserole

- ¼ tsp. rosemary

- ¼ tsp. thyme
- ½ cup mayonnaise
- ½ tsp. dried basil
- ½ tsp. smoked paprika
- 1 cup plain full-fat Greek yogurt
- 1 cup shredded cheese
- 1 tsp. garlic salt
- 1 tsp. onion powder
- 14 oz. bags frozen broccoli
- 8 oz. cream cheese

Directions:

1. Preheat the oven to 350 degrees Fahrenheit and wash your broccoli and cauliflower.
2. Start by placing your cauliflower florets in the blender with raw walnuts, hemp seeds, cumin, garlic powder, onion powder, and salt or a seasoning of your choice.
3. Grind the ingredients together until the mixture you see in your grinder resembles tiny bread crumbs.
4. Place a pan large on the stove and set it to a low temperature and add in 2 tbsp. of avocado oil.

5. While you wait for the pan to heat, place broccoli florets, cream cheese, Greek yogurt, mayonnaise, garlic salt, onion powder, dried basil, smoked paprika, rosemary, and thyme in a large mixing bowl.

6. Now, return to the minced 'meat' and set the temperature on the pan to a medium heat and add in the mixture. Use a spatula or wooden spoon for stirring, and cook 2 to 4 minutes before adding 2 tbsp. adobo sauce.

7. Cook for 5 more minutes; the minced 'meat' should be brown in color and look like browned minced meat. Add in the 2 tbsp. of cheddar cheese.

8. Dish the minced 'meat' into the same mixing bowl as the broccoli, and use a wooden spoon to combine the ingredients.

9. Then grease your casserole dish before dishing the contents of the mixing bowl inside, and drizzle the shredded cheese on top

before transferring the casserole to the already heated oven.

10. Cook the casserole for a maximum of 50 minutes or until the cheese begins to bubble.

11. Remove the dish from the oven, cut into eight equal pieces, dish out the needed amount, serve, and cover and store the rest in the refrigerator.

Cauliflower Broccoli Stir Fry

Cauliflower Broccoli Stir Fry is an amazing dinner meal that is pretty easy to make, and it is another cauliflower and broccoli combo with red bell peppers and mushrooms, which are our keto-friendly vegetables. That just shows you how much you can do when you limit your diet to only nine vegetables.

What you are going to need for this recipe is a frying pan, wooden spoon, and measuring cups and spoons.

The recipe below yields 4 servings for you to absolutely enjoy. You can cover the leftovers and store them in the fridge for later use.

Time: 20 minutes

Serving Size: 1

Prep Time: 10 minutes

Cook Time: 10 minutes

Nutritional Facts/Info:

Calories: 126

Carbs: 8.8 grams

Fat: 7.6 grams

Protein: 4.2 grams

Ingredients:

- ¼ cup soy sauce
- ½ medium red bell pepper
- ½ tsp. red pepper flakes

- 1 medium onion
- 1 tbsp. avocado oil
- 1 tbsp. ginger
- 2 tsp. sesame oil
- 2 whole garlic cloves
- 3 oz. cremini mushrooms
- 4 ounces cauliflower
- 7 oz. broccoli

Directions:

1. Start with washing all your vegetables, then on a cutting board, peel and grate the ginger, mince the garlic, chop the onion, cut the red bell pepper into slices, cut the mushrooms into slices, and break the cauliflower and broccoli into florets (tiny broccoli and cauliflower trees).

2. Place the different ingredients in separate bowls and put every other ingredient aside except for the garlic, ginger, soy sauce, vinegar, and cauliflower florets.

3. Coat the cauliflower florets thoroughly in the garlic, ginger, soy sauce, and vinegar. Allow the

flavors to really sink in by setting the bowl of marinating florets aside.

4. Pour 1 ½ tbsp. of avocado oil into a wok or frying pan that is set on a low-medium heat and throw in onion. The onion should be a light faint brown before you can add in the red bell pepper, mushrooms, and broccoli.

5. Stir the ingredients in the pan together and, once the broccoli and the red bell pepper start to brown, add in the cauliflower and another 1 ½ tbsp. of avocado oil. Note: do not throw away the marinade.

6. Cook the ingredients together for roughly 5 minutes or until the cauliflower browns and pour in the marinade into the wok to be stirred with the ingredients in the pan until the sauces have almost evaporated.

7. Dish the food out into a bowl and dig right in.

Chapter 8: Vegetarian Keto Diet Snack Ideas

Keto Cucumber Sushi

Keto Cucumber Sushi is a cucumber stuffed with other vegetables, so there is no need to worry because there is no fishy business going on here. The snack is crunchy and refreshing and can be used as a side dish.

Time: 20 minutes

Serving Size: 1

Prep Time: 15 minutes

Cook Time: N/A

Nutritional Facts/Info:

Calories: 190

Carbs: 9 grams

Fat: 16 grams

Protein: 1 gram

Ingredients:

- 2 carrots
- 1 cucumber
- 1 tbsp. sriracha
- 1 tsp. soy sauce
- ½ red bell pepper
- ½ yellow bell pepper
- ⅓ cup mayonnaise
- ¼ avocado

Directions:

1. In a small bowl, whisk the mayonnaise, sriracha, and soy sauce to make the dipping sauce, then put the sauce in the fridge.
2. The next thing to do is cut your

avocado, carrots, and bell peppers into slices.

3. Cut your cucumber in two and use a teaspoon to hollow out the center. Use a butter knife to spread avocado around the inside of the cucumber.

4. Stuff the cucumber with bell peppers and carrots until the cucumber is packed with the vegetables.

5. Lastly, slice the cucumber into one-inch thick pieces and enjoy with the sauce.

Avocado 'Potato' Chip

Avocado 'Potato' Chip is another one of those weird sounding recipes, but it is really not. This is a salty, healthy, and enjoyable snack that even your friends might be interested in. You can store the leftovers in a jar in the pantry or a sealable bag in the pantry.

The recipe yields 16 chips.

Time: 45 minutes

Serving Size: 1

Prep Time: 10 minutes

Cook Time: 35 minutes

Nutritional Facts/Info:

Calories: 120

Carbs: 4 grams

Fat: 10 grams

Protein: 7 grams

Ingredients:

- ½ tsp. garlic
- ½ tsp. Italian seasoning
- ¾ cup freshly grated Parmesan
- 1 large ripe avocado
- 1 tsp. lemon juice
- Salt and pepper

Directions:

1. Start by preheating your oven to

325 degrees Fahrenheit.

2. Cut the avocado in two, dish it into a medium bowl, and mash the avocado with a fork until it is smooth in texture.

3. Add the Parmesan, lemon juice, garlic powder, basil, oregano, rosemary, and salt. Lay parchment paper on the baking sheet.

4. Use a teaspoon to place the mixture on the baking sheet and space out. Use the teaspoon to flat the scoop.

5. Bake for 30 minutes and wait for the chips to cool before digging in.

Strawberry Milkshake

Strawberry Milkshake is another one of the great treats you can make with keto-friendly fruit like strawberries. You can enjoy this recipe as a snack or dessert.

Every sip is cooling and sweet but keto-friendly nonetheless.

The majority of the fats (21.47 grams), carbs (1.63 grams), and protein (1.69 grams) comes from the ¼ cup of heavy whipping cream.

The recipe yields only 1 serving; try not to overindulge.

Time: 5 minutes

Serving Size: 1 glass

Prep Time: 3 minutes

Cook Time: 2 minutes

Nutritional Facts/Info:

Calories: 368

Carbs: 2.42 grams

Fat: 38.85 grams

Protein: 1.69 grams

Ingredients:

- 7 ice cubes

- 2 tbsp. sugar-free strawberry Torani (or sugar-free strawberry syrup)
- 1 tbsp. MCT oil
- ¾ cup coconut milk (from the carton)
- ¼ tsp. xanthan gum
- ¼ cup heavy cream

Directions:

1. Start blending the 7 ice cubes in the blender.
2. When the ice is crushed pour in your syrup, MCT oil, milk, xanthan gum, and heavy cream and blend the ingredients together until smooth and soft pink in color.
3. Serve in a tall glass and prepare to have your taste buds lose their tiny minds!

Mixed Berries Fruit Roll Ups

Mixed Berries Fruit Roll Ups are the ideal snack time idea. Growing up with fruit roll ups and dried fruit, this recipe was exciting for me to make, and you are seriously going to love these.

You can try the recipe with other keto-friendly fruits or the ones that are low enough in carbs to try out; you know, the fruits you should only enjoy occasionally.

Nevertheless, what you are going to need for this recipe is a strainer, a spoon, a bowl, a silicone mat, and a baking pan. You are going to use an oven to dry out your fruit roll up, but if you have a dehydrator, you can use that too.

The recipe below produces 8 pieces of fruity fruit roll ups.

Time: 5 hours 15 minutes

Serving Size: 1

Prep Time: 15 minutes

Cook Time: 5 hours

Nutritional Facts/Info:

Calories: 14

Carbs: 7.5 grams

Fat: 0.2 grams

Protein: 0.3 grams

Ingredients:

- 1 tbsp. lemon juice
- 3 tbsp. erythritol
- 1 cup raspberries
- 1 cup strawberries

Directions:

1. Start with washing your raspberries and strawberries, then cut the stem of your strawberries and cut each strawberry into four pieces.
2. You are going to purée your berries into a bowl with a strainer and large spoon, although if you've got a blender or food processor, then you can use those, but our process purées and

removes the seeds from the berries at the same time.

3. Place the chopped strawberries in the strainer, let the strainer hover over a small- to medium-sized bowl, and press the strawberries until all the juices have been drained out.

4. Now, rinse out the strawberry seeds from your strainer and now purée the raspberries in the same way you did with the strawberries. You can cut the raspberries if you think it will make things easier.

5. Once both berries have been puréed into the same bowl, add in the erythritol and 1 tbsp. of lemon juice. Stir the ingredients together until fully combined.

6. Proceed by turning on your oven and setting the temperature to 140 degrees Fahrenheit.

7. Place a silicone mat on your baking pan, gently pour the pure on the mat, and use a clean spoon to even it out, and then cook it in

the oven for 3 to 5 hours. When it is ready, the center of the dried purée should not be sticky.

8. You should carefully peel the fruit roll up from the silicone and cut it into the shape and number of pieces you want, or cut eight strips out and roll them up and secure them with tape.

9. Note that the fruit roll up will be dry but will get sticky overnight, so be sure not to place them too close together in case they stick to one another.

10. You can enjoy the roll ups after they have completely set (i.e., gotten sticky).

Low Carb Pumpkin Spice Fat Bombs

This recipe is ideal for individuals on-the-go and those who would not be able to live without the taste of pumpkin spice. You will be able to meet your fat intake needs with these little treats.

You are sure to have fun making these and can either use a candy mold, ice cube tray, or a baking tray, the latter of which is what we used in the recipe below.

The recipe below yields 12 servings.

Time: 3 hours 10 minutes

Serving Size: 1

Prep Time: 10 minutes

Cook Time: 3 hours

Nutritional Facts/Info:

Calories: 137

Carbs: 1.4 grams

Fat: 14.1 grams

Protein: 1.2 grams

Ingredients:

- 4 oz. cream cheese
- 2 tsp. pumpkin spice
- ½ cup pecans
- ½ cup butter
- ½ cup pumpkin purée
- ¼ cup powdered erythritol

Directions:

1. Start by placing your butter and cream cheese in a microwave-safe bowl and allow the two ingredients to soften in the microwave for 30 to 45 seconds, and then mix them together until light yellow and creamy in color and texture.

2. Now, pour the pumpkin purée into the bowl of butter and cheese and combine the ingredients until a darker shade of yellow is formed and the mixture is creamy in texture.

3. Proceed by stirring the powdered erythritol and pumpkin spice into the same mixture; the color and texture should still be the same as above.

4. Place some parchment or wax paper onto your baking tray before pouring the fully combined mixture onto the parchment paper. Smooth out the top of the mixture with a non-stick spoon. Ensure the mixture is 1 inch thick in height.

5. Sprinkle on your pecans, being sure that they sink just enough into the mixture, before putting the baking tray in the freezer for a maximum time of 3 hours.

6. Once the 3 hours are done, you can remove the baking tray from the freezer and proceed by heating the blade of your knife in hot water, which should make it easier to cut the mold, before cutting the fat bomb mold into 12 even pieces or even smaller pieces if that is what you prefer.

Portobello Mushroom Fries

Portobello Mushroom Fries are the perfect snack to have on the weekend when you just want to enjoy tender fries covered in melted cheese and tasty spices, and you are allowed to substitute the cheese and spices mentioned in the recipe for your own spices and cheese preferences.

Additional notes:

- For added crunch, color, and flavor, you can add chopped scallions or red bell pepper to the recipes. You can add one of these or both on top of the cheese before you melt the cheese in the oven.

The recipe below yields 2 servings of fries and tastes better straight out of the oven; therefore, if you only want to make one serving, then halve the ingredients.

Time: 25 minutes

Serving Size: 1

Prep Time: 15 minutes

Cook Time: 10 minutes

Nutritional Facts/Info:

Calories: 119.5

Carbs: 4.2 grams

Fat: 12.97 grams

Protein: 31.93 grams

Ingredients:

- 2 large Portobello mushroom caps
- 1 large egg
- 1 tbsp. dried chives
- ½ cup shredded Parmesan cheese
- ½ tsp. garlic powder
- ½ tsp. smoked paprika
- ¼ tsp. cayenne pepper
- ¼ cup shredded cheddar cheese

Directions:

1. Preheat the oven to 425 degrees Fahrenheit.
2. After that, start by washing your mushrooms before placing them on a cutting board.
3. Once the mushrooms are on the board, cut them into thick slices; they should resemble the shape of French fries.
4. Now, in a small bowl, mix together the Parmesan cheese, cheddar cheese, smoked paprika, dried chives, and cayenne pepper. Ensure that both of the cheese is thinly shredded.
5. Set the bowl of cheese and spices aside before lining your baking tray with some and then bring out a shallow dish.
6. Whisk your egg together in the shallow dish with garlic powder and another seasoning of your choice and coat the mushroom slices in the eggy mix. Then lay the coated slices out on the baking tray and put the tray in the oven, allowing the slices to

bake for a maximum of 10 minutes.

7. Remove the tray from the oven and cover the mushroom fries in the cheese and spice mixture before putting the tray back in the oven for another 5 minutes.

8. Once the cheese has melted, you can remove the tray from the oven, dish out the fries, and enjoy right away.

Avocado & Goat Cheese Bites

Avocado & Goat Cheese Bites are a colorful snack that combines the wonderful tastes of avocado, radicchio lettuce, and goat cheese. The snack only takes 15 minutes to make and is ideally low in both carbs and calories.

The recipe below makes 16 little enjoyable bites that are best stored in an airtight container in your fridge, and it should contain the freshness of the ingredients for a maximum of 2 days.

Time: 15 minutes

Serving Size: 1

Prep Time: 15 minutes

Cook Time: N/A

Nutritional Facts/Info:

Calories: 91

Carbs: 0.9 grams

Fat: 7.5 grams

Protein: 4.7 grams

Ingredients:

- 1 large avocado
- 8 oz. goat cheese, softened
- 2 cloves garlic, grated
- 3.9 oz. radicchio lettuce

- 1 tbsp. oregano
- 1 tbsp. rosemary
- 1 tbsp. basil
- 1 tbsp. kosher salt
- 1 tbsp. black pepper

Directions:

1. Start by cutting the stem off the bottom of the radicchio lettuce. Collect 16 fresh medium-sized leaves from the lettuce, and store the remains in a tightly sealed container for other near-future recipes.
2. Thoroughly wash the leaves, then lay them out on a cutting board or kitchen tray to dry while you grate the garlic cloves, and then put the grated garlic in a medium-sized bowl.
3. Sprinkle the oregano, rosemary, basil, salt, and pepper; mix in the softened goat cheese until the ingredients in the bowl resemble a white chunky paste.
4. Next, you need to cut the large avocado into 16 thick slices, cut

each slice in 2, place 2 smaller slices on a radicchio leaf, and scoop 1 tbsp. of the goat cheese mix onto the avocado.

5. Repeat the above process with the other leaves and then you can serve and enjoy.

Chapter 9: Vegetarian Keto Dessert Ideas

Blackberry Pudding

Blackberry Pudding is an amazing after-dinner dish. The dessert is light and fluffy and sweet to the taste. You will seriously enjoy this dish, so we recommend that you do not overindulge.

This recipe yields 2 servings.

Time: 35 minutes

Serving Size: 1

Prep Time: 10 minutes

Cook Time: 25 minutes

Nutritional Facts/Info:

Calories: 459.5

Carbs: 4.91 grams

Fat: 44.04 grams

Protein: 9.1 grams

Ingredients:

- ¼ cup blackberries
- ¼ cup coconut flour
- ¼ tsp. baking powder
- 1 lemon (zested)
- 10 drops liquid Stevia
- 2 tablespoons erythritol
- 2 tbsp. butter
- 2 tbsp. coconut oil
- 2 tbsp. heavy cream
- 2 tsp. lemon juice
- 5 large egg yolks

Directions:

1. Turn on the oven and set the temperature to 350 degrees Fahrenheit.
2. You will need two small dishes and a spoon to separate the yolks from the egg whites: break the

egg inside one bowl, then spoon out the egg yolk and transfer the yolk to the second bowl. Repeat the action with the remaining four eggs.

3. You can cover and put away the bowl of egg whites in your fridge, and use them for an egg-white veggie breakfast the next day.

4. Whisk the egg yolks together, then add the erythritol and liquid Stevia, and whisk together until fully combined.

5. Next, add the lemon juice, the zest of one lemon, heavy cream, coconut oil, and the butter. Stir the ingredients together until mixed.

6. Now, add the coconut flour and baking powder to the bowl and mix until fully combined. The mixture is slightly thick and bright yellow in color.

7. Add blackberries to the mix before scooping the mixture into two oven-safe small bowls, and bake in the oven for 20 minutes.

8. Allow the pudding to cool and it should be slightly liquefied on the inside and the top of the pudding should be brown on the sides.
9. Serve and enjoy as is.

Coconut Chip Cookies

Coconut Chip Cookies are a craving-combating kind of cookie. They are not only crunchy and chewy but they are also healthy and keto-friendly. It does not mean you can overindulge, but you sure can enjoy them every now and again.

The recipe below yields 16 cookies.

Time: 35 minutes

Serving Size: 1 cookie

Prep Time: 10 minutes

Cook Time: 25 minutes

Nutritional Facts/Info:

Calories: 192.38

Carbs: 2.17 grams

Fat: 17.44 grams

Protein: 4.67 grams

Ingredients:

- 20 drops liquid Stevia
- 2 large eggs
- 1 cup almond flour
- ½ cup cacao nibs
- ½ cup unsweetened coconut flakes
- ½ almond butter
- ⅓ erythritol
- ¼ cup melted butter
- ¼ tsp. salt
- 1 tsp. vanilla extract

Directions:

1. Turn the oven on and set the temperature to 350 degrees Fahrenheit.

2. Begin by setting out the required ingredients, measuring cups, and a medium bowl for mixing.

3. In a microwaveable cup, melt the butter for 30 seconds in the microwave, and then pour the melted butter into the mixing bowl.

4. Whisk the butter for a second before adding the almond butter, eggs, liquid Stevia, and vanilla extract.

5. Once the wet ingredients are properly combined, the mixture should be coffee brown in color and not too watery.

6. You are going to add, then stir, add, then stir the dry ingredients, one by one. Start with the cacao nibs, then almond flour, coconut flakes, erythritol, and add the salt last. The mixture should be soft, doughy, and brown when properly combined.

7. Now, lay out some wax paper on your baking tray or use a non-stick spray if you do not have wax

paper, and use a spoon to scoop out and evenly flatten out 16 cookies on the tray.

8. Bake the cookies for 25 minutes or until the sides begin to brown. Once you take the cookies out of the oven, allow them to cool before serving.

Peanut Butter Balls

Peanut Butter Balls are a quick and simple dessert or snack to make, and it satisfies any cravings you may have. When it comes to storing you can keep these in the fridge.

The recipe yields 15 Coconut Peanut Butter Balls.

Time: 3 hours 10 minutes

Serving Size: 1

Prep Time: 10 minutes

Cook Time: 3 hours

Nutritional Facts/Info:

Calories: 35.13

Carbs: 1.51 grams

Fat: 3.19 grams

Protein: 0.98 grams

Ingredients:

- ½ cup unsweetened shredded coconut
- 2 ½ tsp. powdered erythritol
- 2 tsp. almond flour
- 3 tbsp. creamy peanut butter
- 3 tsp. unsweetened cocoa powder

Directions:

1. Start by whisking the peanut butter in the mixing bowl for 15 to 20 seconds.
2. Then add in the cocoa powder and beat together until smooth and brown in color, and then mix

in the erythritol and the almond flour.

3. Once the mixture is combined, it should resemble a browned peanut butter. Now, place the mix in the freezer for 1 hour.

4. The mixture should be firm and you can use a teaspoon to scoop and measure the size of the balls, and then mold them with your hands before dumping them in a bowl of shredded coconut.

5. Place the balls back in the freezer for 1 to 2 hours to set before serving.

Frosty

Absolutely the best dessert idea yet and is totally capable of curing your ice-cream craving, and is not too sweet. The recipe yields four servings. You can store the remains in the freezer, and allow it to sit aside if it happens to be completely frozen.

Time: 50 minutes

Serving Size: 4

Prep Time: 15 minutes

Cook Time: 35 minutes

Nutritional Facts/Info:

Calories: 164

Carbs: 14.1 grams

Fat: 17 grams

Protein: 1.4 grams

Ingredients:

- 2 tbsp. cocoa powder
- 3 tbsp. erythritol
- 1 tsp. vanilla extract
- 1 ½ cup heavy whipping cream
- A pinch of salt

Directions:

1. Use a large bowl to whisk together the cream, cocoa, erythritol, vanilla, and salt.
2. Dish the mixture into a sealable bag and store in the freezer for 35 minutes.
3. The mixture should be just frozen when you pull it out of the freezer, at which point you cut a corner piece of the plastic bag, and squeeze the mixture into a tall glass or bowl.
4. Serve and enjoy.

Low-Carb Carrot Cake

Low-Carb Carrot Cake can be keto-friendly if made correctly, but if you do not trust your baking abilities, then substitute the carrot with zucchini instead, which is equally as tasty and twice as satisfying.

Other things to note about the recipe:

- You can use sunflower seed flour instead of almond flour.
- You do not have to use pecans in this recipe.
- Do not replace the sweetener in this recipe with a liquid sweetener.
- Your safest bet with this recipe is to grate the carrot yourself and not use grated carrots from a bag.

The recipe below yields 8 slices that you can store in the fridge for a period of 3 days in a tightly sealed container to ensure the cake does not dry out.

Time: 40 minutes

Serving Size: 1 slice

Prep Time: 15 minutes

Cook Time: 20 minutes

Nutritional Facts/Info:

Calories: 387

Carbs: 4.7 grams

Fat: 35.6 grams

Protein: 9.7 grams

Ingredients:

- 7 tbsp. butter
- 4 large eggs
- 4 oz. cream cheese
- 2 tbsp. cinnamon powder
- 1 tsp. vanilla extract
- 1 tbsp. heavy cream
- 1 tbsp. baking powder
- ¾ cup erythritol
- ½ tsp. ginger powder
- ½ nutmeg powder
- ½ cup pecans
- 1.5 cups almond flour
- 1 large carrot

Directions:

1. Start by turning on your oven to 350 degrees Fahrenheit, getting your baking tray out, and putting wax paper on the baking sheet.
2. Then, in a small bowl, you will make your cream cheese frosting by whisking together the softened

4 oz. of cream cheese, 2 tbsp. of butter, 1 tsp. of vanilla extract, 1 tbsp. of heavy cream, and ¼ cup powdered erythritol until smooth and creamy.

3. Place the bowl of cream cheese frosting in the fridge for later use.

4. Proceed by chopping your pecans into pieces, and then put them aside.

5. Now, in a large bowl, combine the melted remaining 5 tbsp. of butter and the remaining ½ cup of erythritol and whisk these ingredients together until smooth.

6. Whisk in the 4 eggs before stirring in the baking powder, cinnamon, ginger, nutmeg, and vanilla extract.

7. Finally, pour in the chopped pecans, almond flour, and your grated carrot into the same bowl and combine the ingredients until oat-like in color and texture.

8. Pour the mixture into the baking tray lined with wax paper,

smooth out with a spoon, and bake in the oven for 20 minutes. (You can test the readiness of the cake by sticking a tooth-pick or fork in the center of the cake; if the tooth-pick or fork comes back clean, then the cake is ready.)

9. Once the cake has been baked, allow the cake to cool for about 10 to 15 minutes, then layer the top of the cake in cream cheese frosting, cut into eight pieces, and serve or store for later enjoyment.

Low-Carb Chia Pudding

Yes, another pudding, but this has to be the most creative dessert recipe yet.

This low-carb dessert could even work as an enjoyable breakfast meal. You could add some strawberries and other keto-friendly fruit like cantaloupe as a topping to really make the recipe your own.

The recipe below yields 3 servings.

Time: 25 minutes

Serving Size: 1 short glass

Prep Time: 25 minutes

Cook Time: N/A

Nutritional Facts/Info:

Calories: 187.07

Carbs: 4.53 grams

Fat: 11.47 grams

Protein: 6.27 grams

Ingredients:

- 2 tsp. unsweetened cocoa powder
- 2 tbsp. monk fruit sweetener
- 1 tsp. vanilla extract
- 1 ½ cups unsweetened almond milk
- ½ cup chia seeds

- 4 strawberries

Directions:

1. First, gather all the above-mentioned ingredients along with any other keto-friendly fruits you want to add to the dessert recipe. (Be sure to check your macros, specifically your intake of carbs for this meal and what you consume the rest of the day to ensure you are not kicked out of ketosis.)

2. In a large bowl, stir together the chia seeds, unsweetened almond milk, monk fruit sweetener, and vanilla extract. Place the bowl in the fridge for 20 minutes.

3. During the 20 minutes, gather your strawberries, cut each strawberry in four, and use a sifter and large spoon to purée the strawberries into a small bowl.

4. Once the 20 minutes have passed, bring out two more other bowls, divide the chia seed mix into

three bowls (the two bowls you brought out and the one bowl with the strawberry purée).

5. Pour the strawberry and chia mix evenly into your dessert glasses once you have combined the two recipes.

6. Add unsweetened cocoa powder to the second bowl of chia seed mix and, once you have fully combined the ingredients, pour them evenly into the same three glasses you did the strawberry chia.

7. The last bowl is vanilla and does not need to be combined with anything else, so add that to the glasses, and top the dessert with heavy cream or keto-friendly fruit and enjoy.

Peanut Butter Chocolate Cups

Peanut Butter Chocolate Cups are the treat that curb both your peanut butter and possible chocolate cravings. You can store these for three weeks in the fridge and for 3 months in the freezer. Although, if you are going to store them in the freezer, allow them to 'cool' outside of the freezer for 15 minutes before consumption (to allow for the chocolate to soften a bit and make eating easier).

Additional notes:

- You are going to need cupcake molds.
- You can substitute the peanut butter for keto-friendly seed butter if you wish to avoid nuts.
- Another substitution you can make is to use coconut oil in the place of butter.
- We use sugar-free plain peanut butter but you can use a keto-friendly alternative.
- As for the chocolate, stick to a sugar-free and low-carb chocolate.

The recipe below yields 8 chocolate peanut butter cups.

Time: 50 minutes

Serving Size: 1

Prep Time: 30 minutes

Cook Time: 20 minutes

Nutritional Facts/Info:

Calories: 204.9

Carbs: 3.4 grams

Fat: 19.3 grams

Protein: 4.1 grams

Ingredients:

- 4 oz. low-carb milk chocolate
- ½ tsp. vanilla extract
- ½ cup peanut butter
- ⅓ cup erythritol powder
- ¼ cup butter

Directions:

1. Start by placing your silicone cupcake molds in your cupcake tray.
2. Continue by placing a sauce pan on the stove and set the temperature to a low-medium heat.
3. Scoop the butter into the saucepan and stir until smooth, then stir in the powdered erythritol, peanut butter, and vanilla extract until the mixture is creamy and brown in texture and color.
4. Pour the mixture into the silicone molds and place the cupcake tray in the freezer for 15 minutes.
5. During the 15 minutes, pour some water into a small pot, place the temperature on a medium heat and let the water boil before placing a bowl wide enough to fit over the opening on the pot. Set the temperature to a low heat.
6. Pour your chocolate into the bowl and stir together with a whisk until the chocolate is smooth and

creamy, and once the 15 minutes have passed, remove the peanut butter molds from the freezer.

7. Allow the chocolate to cool slightly, as you don't want to melt your peanut butter molds. Once cooled, pour the chocolate out evenly between the 8 molds.

8. Lastly, put the tray back in the freezer for 15 minutes, then remove before carefully removing the peanut butter cups from their molds, and you can enjoy right away and store the rest in a tightly sealed container.

Conclusion

There are three main aspects you learned about in this guide and they are how to:

#1. Effectively Lose Weight on the Ketogenic Diet

The ketogenic diet is a low-carb, high-fat, and moderate-protein diet. When there are no carbs in the body to be burnt for energy, the body defaults to using fat for fuel. When the body has this metabolic reaction, we call it ketosis. However, we do not only lose weight on the ketogenic diet because of what we eat but also from how we choose to eat (our number of meals) and how many calories we choose to consume all together. The key aspects are the high fat and low carb components and how this forces your body to burn both the fat from the food you eat plus your body fat for fuel. A vegetarian ketogenic diet should be always combined with regular exercise and watching your calories.

#2. Adopt Healthier Eating Habits

The ketogenic diet and the vegetarian diet both promote healthy eating habits, the former encourages you to eat fewer carbs and consume more healthy fats, and the latter encourages you to stick to a diet that comprises mostly fruits and vegetables. These diets make you conscious of what foods are around you at all times, therefore, over time you eventually develop healthy eating habits because you are made more aware of what you are putting into your body.

#3. Improve on Vegetarian Recipes

The vegetarian-ketogenic combo diet really allows for creative and fun recipes for you to try out. Think of a vegetarian recipe that isn't keto-friendly and think of a way to make it keto-friendly, then add it to your weekly meal plan.

We truly hope this guide has been helpful to you and that you will be able to implement a vegetarian keto diet effectively in your own life. Remember that everything takes time and patience, and you should remain fully determined and focused, and not let any excuse or worry stand in the way of you making the changes you want to see in your life.

Use our guide as a reference when you get started on the ketogenic diet; we believe that this reference will be effective and that the comprehensive chapters have taught you all you need and have wanted to learn about the vegetarian ketogenic diet.

Do Not Go Yet; One Last Thing To Do
If you enjoyed this book or found it useful,
I'd be very grateful if you'd post a short
review on Amazon. Your support does make
a difference, and I read all the reviews
personally so I can get your feedback and
make this book even better.

Thanks again for your support!

Printed in Great Britain
by Amazon